FACIAL FEMINIZATION SURGERY

The Journey to Gender Affirmation

SECOND EDITION

Jordan Deschamps-Braly, M.D., F.A.C.S.

Douglas Ousterhout, M.D., D.D.S., F.A.C.S.

Addicus Books

Omaha, Nebraska

AN ADDICUS NONFICTION BOOK

———

ISBN 978-1-950091-39-3

Cover design and typography by Peri Gabriel Design

This book is not intended to serve as a substitute for a physician. Nor is it the authors' intent
to give medical advice contrary to that of an attending physician.

LIBRARY OF CONGRESS
CATALOGING-IN-PUBLICATION DATA

———

Names: Deschamps-Braly, Jordan, 1979, author. | Ousterhout, Douglas K., author.

Title: Facial feminization surgery : the journey to gender affirmation / Jordan Deschamps-Braly, M.D., F.A.C.S.,
Douglas K. Ousterhout, M.D., D.D.S.

Description: Second [edition]. | Omaha, Nebraska : Addicus Books Inc. [2021] | Revision of:
Facial feminization surgery / Douglas K. Ousterhout.

Identifiers: LCCN 2020031902 (print) | LCCN 2020031903 (ebook) | ISBN 9781950091393 (trade paperback) |
ISBN 9781950091478 (pdf) | ISBN 9781950091485 (epub) | ISBN 9781950091492 (kindle edition)

Subjects: LCSH: Face—Surgery. | Surgery, Plastic. | Transfeminine individuals.

Classification: LCC RD119.5.F33 O96 2021 (print) | LCC RD119.5.F33 (ebook) | DDC 617.5/20592—dc23

LC record available at https://lccn.loc.gov/2020031902
LC ebook record available at https://lccn.loc.gov/2020031903

2009035951

Addicus Books, Inc.
P.O. Box 45327
Omaha, Nebraska 68145
AddicusBooks.com

Printed in the United States of America

10 9 8 7 6 5 4 3 2 1

To my mentors—great surgeons all:

Douglas Ousterhout, Daniel Marchac, Joachim Obwegeser,

Arlen Denny, and Christian El Amm

To my parents George Braly and Dania Deschamps-Braly

—JORDAN DESCHAMPS-BRALY M.D.

———

To Naomi and Ken
Nancy
Dean and Don
Don, Susan, Oliver, Thomas, Lauren
Marlene
Jessica, Michaela, and Sarah

—DOUGLAS K. OUSTERHOUT, M.D., D.D.S.

———

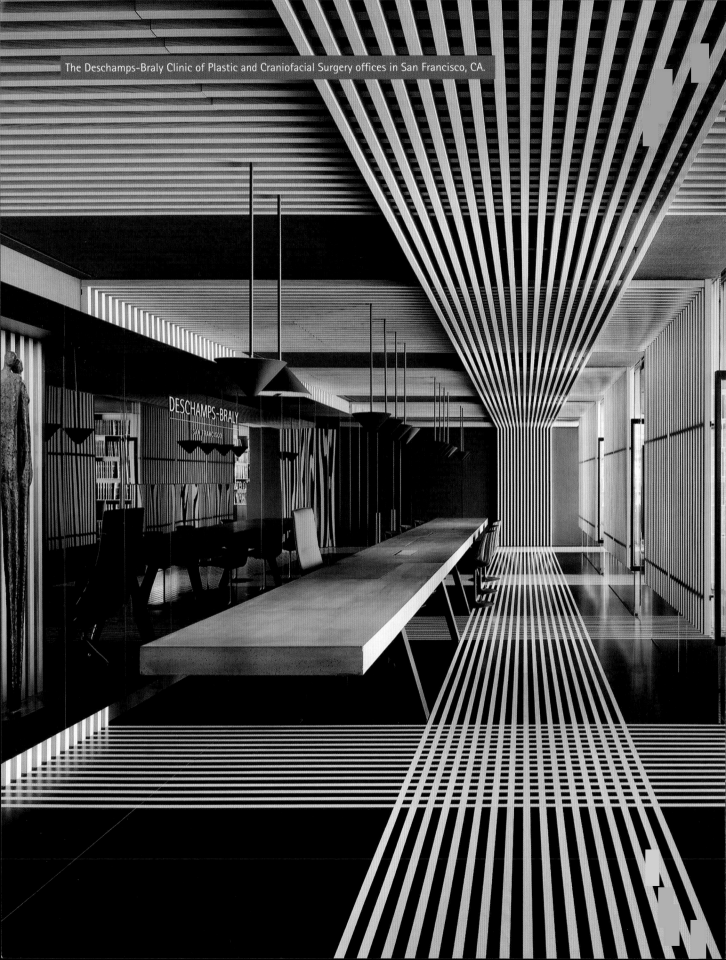
The Deschamps-Braly Clinic of Plastic and Craniofacial Surgery offices in San Francisco, CA.

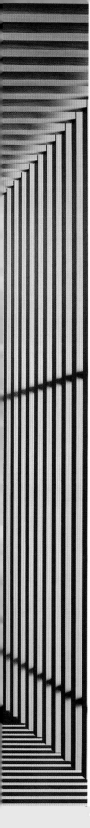

Contents

═══

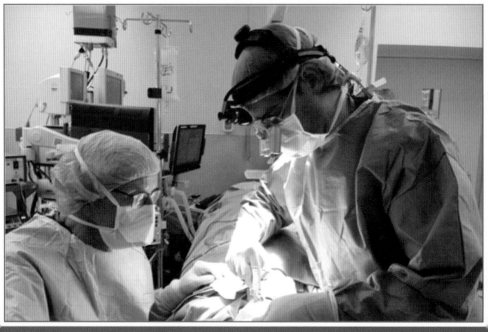
Dr. Deschamps-Braly and Dr. Ousterhout performing facial feminization surgery.

Acknowledgments

MY STORY BEGINS WITH "DOUGLAS"— Dr. Ousterhout. His pioneering work in aesthetic surgery of the craniofacial skeleton evolved into procedures that changed the lives of many transgender people. For these patients, gender incongruence was a terrible fact of daily life. Dr. O felt strongly that his work and expertise should be passed on and continued—hopefully, in hands as skillful as his own. When I first performed surgery with Dr. O, I was impressed with his deftness, focus, and stamina. While he was more than twice my age, he could ably perform procedures that typically took ten to twelve hours.

At the end of the summer of 2014, Dr. Ousterhout "retired" from active surgery. Some surgeons wait too long to make that decision. Dr. Ousterhout retired while his skills were still razor sharp at the age of seventy-nine. I was then extremely fortunate to have Dr. Ousterhout in the operating room as my assistant on a regular basis. After several years, he settled into "full" retirement. While semiretired, he taught me the techniques, visual understanding, and judgment required to perform these complex, magnificent surgeries.

As we collaborated on many surgeries, I learned the skill and knowledge needed for facial feminization from a great teacher, mentor, and friend.

Douglas never showed or taught anyone else how to do this work. He rejected several surgeons who approached him as being inadequately trained and skilled. He felt strongly that one had to be not only a plastic surgeon, but also an accomplished craniofacial and maxillofacial surgeon to do this work. To train me as his successor, he required that I spend several years working with him. He would not allow casual "visitors" in the operating room who he worried would learn just enough to be "dangerous."

Other great surgeons have helped me lay the foundation for doing this work. Dr. Arlen Denny at Children's Hospital, Wisconsin (who, like Dr. Ousterhout, trained with Dr. Paul Tessier in Paris) taught me to perform complex pediatric craniofacial surgeries during a yearlong fellowship. After my training in Europe and my move to San Francisco, Arlen introduced me to Dr. Ousterhout. For that, I will always be grateful.

The late Dr. Daniel Marchac and Dr. Eric Arnaud, both in Paris, provided me with an enormous opportunity to further my skills in craniofacial surgery. With their guidance I was able to acquire a wealth of experience in aesthetic facial surgery. That year of surgery in Paris was an opportunity and experience unlike any other available to American surgeons, even at the most prestigious institutions in North America. Dr. Marchac passed away shortly after my time in Paris. I was truly blessed to be the last young surgeon to have had this great experience with Dr. Marchac.

Dr. Obwegeser of Zurich, Switzerland, also trained me in one of the many essential skills for facial feminization surgery—orthognathic (jaw) surgery.

Finally, I want to express my appreciation to Doug Ousterhout for selecting me to continue performing his pioneering surgeries, and for "showing me the ropes."

To each of these mentors, I express my enormous gratitude.

—JORDAN DESCHAMPS-BRALY, M.D.

Foreword

IN 1995, DR. DOUGLAS OUSTERHOUT mailed me his brochure about facial feminization. It contained a life-changing epiphany. It began: "Looking feminine is, of course, extremely important to you. First impressions are often based just upon your face. That which is first seen in an initial contact is frequently what defines you."

Dr. O then described exactly why my forehead seemed to be my main hindrance to having a feminine face. I had previously undergone an expensive yet useless hair transplant that did nothing to address the underlying structural issues. Dr. O gave me the language to describe what I knew I needed. His brochure mentioned his ground-breaking book *Aesthetic Contouring of the Craniofacial Skeleton,* which I then read in one sitting at my alma mater's medical library.

My results in 1996, from Dr. O's work, literally changed my life. Against my better judgment, I posted his before and after photos of me online to help others. Dr. O got very busy after that.

My advocacy of the triad of facial hair removal, facial feminization, and voice, led to a shift in priorities for many transwomen's transition timelines. At the time, medical options focused on the so-called "triadic therapies": a lengthy *real-life test (RLT),* followed by *hormone replacement therapy (HRT),* followed by *sex reassignment surgery (SRS).* Access to all were tightly controlled through medical gatekeeping. Meanwhile, the informed consent model that governed most plastic surgery was already the prevailing model in maxillofacial and craniofacial surgery for transwomen.

Following her own excellent results with Dr. O, my friend Lynn Conway quickly became an enthusiastic evangelist as well. She suggested using the acronym *FFS* for *facial feminization surgery,* to elevate its importance to the level of HRT and SRS.

Twenty years after I wrote to Dr. O, his handpicked successor Jordan Deschamps-Braly, M.D., sent me a lovely email of introduction, updating me on their plans for

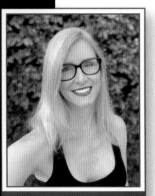

Andrea James

the next generation of world-class plastic and craniofacial surgery for our community.

It quickly became clear that Dr. O's decade-long search for a successor led him to the perfect choice. Dr. D, as he is known to a new generation of grateful patients, has already made many innovations of his own, including significant reductions in procedure times and updated terminology such as "facial gender confirmation surgery." Dr. D also offers a suite of procedures tailored for a wider range of ethnicities and gender identities and what can only be described as impeccable taste and artistry.

Dr. D has established himself as the surgeon of choice for those who expect the best results and service. His gorgeous office itself is worth a trip to San Francisco. His training, deep concern for his patients, and remarkable results, have set him apart in what has become a major specialty field since I posted my results online a quarter century ago.

Facial feminization surgery remains the best investment I have ever made in my life. It pays off with every face-to-face interaction I've had since then. It has helped me with jobs, dates, film roles, and respect. I move through the world more confidently and safely because of it. I urge you to make the trip to Dr. D's office, as an investment in yourself and your future.

— ANDREA JAMES
Filmmaker and Consumer Activist

Introduction

IT IS DIFFICULT TO EXPRESS the profound joy I have felt working with the transgender community. Some of my greatest professional and personal moments have been in meeting male-to-female individuals and hearing their compelling stories.

Yet, my most memorable and rewarding experiences have been in helping individuals transition from birth gender to new gender. I'm proud to say that the facial feminization surgeries I perfected have produced incredible changes in physical appearances and self-esteem for hundreds of transgender individuals.

How did my journey into this field begin? For twenty-five years, I was the senior surgeon at the Center for Craniofacial Anomalies at the University of California, San Francisco (UCSF). There, I frequently collaborated with a great neurosurgeon to correct the malformed or damaged skulls of children. I left the university in 1998, to devote 80 percent of my practice time to the care of transgender people.

In my book *Aesthetic Contouring of the Craniofacial Skeleton,* I provided other surgeons with a guide for changing the size of the facial skeleton. Decreasing the size was the best way to feminize the faces of male-to-female individuals. The reason? The facial features of a man need to be smaller to look like the profile of a woman.

This book attempts to explain many of the facial feminization procedures we use for transgender individuals in language you can understand. It is a consumer guide for anyone contemplating and/or planning facial feminization surgery. Achieving the best aesthetic results may also require procedures that have nothing to do with feminization. So, we have devoted several chapters to topics such as augmenting the cheeks and temple and repositioning the upper and lower jaws.

There are also chapters on rhytidectomies, blepharoplasties, and otoplasties—surgeries that you may want to consider. Designed to lift your face, renew your

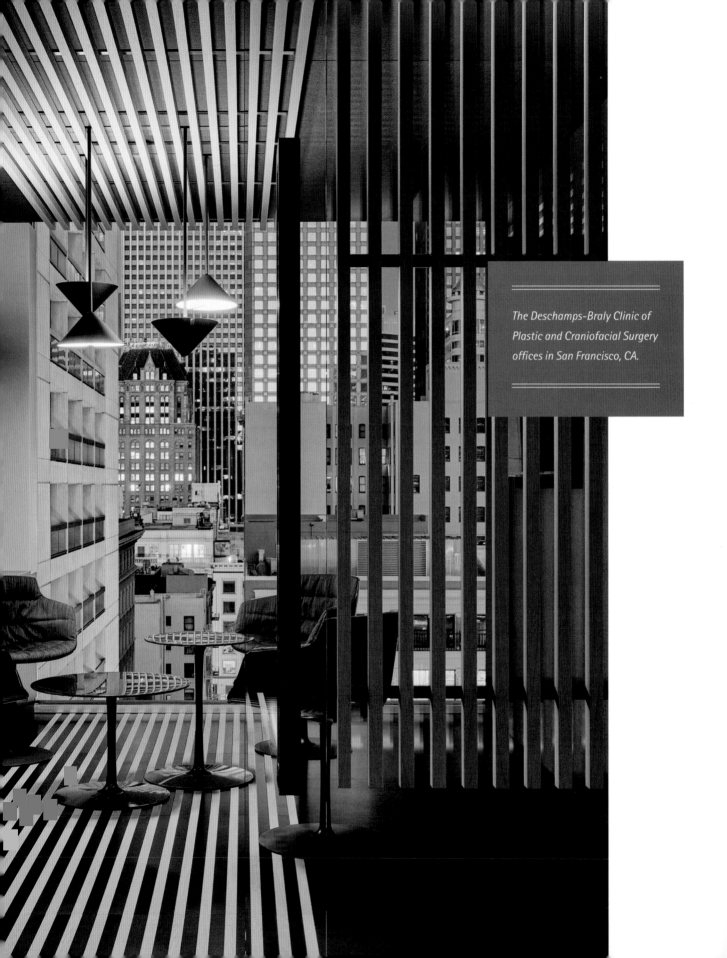

The Deschamps-Braly Clinic of Plastic and Craniofacial Surgery offices in San Francisco, CA.

eyes, or reduce your ears, these surgeries will revitalize your looks. Improving the appearance of your teeth and hair is also very important and is discussed.

This book does not cover other procedures for leaving your birth gender and taking on a new gender. It does not address gender confirmation surgery of the genitals and chest (GRS/GCS) or aesthetic surgeries for areas other than the face.

Our goal is to advise you about which procedures will produce the best facial outcome for you. We hope that you use the information to evaluate the validity of your doctor's suggestions and make informed decisions about undergoing facial surgery.

The opinions expressed in this book are ours alone and are based on our combined experience of completing thousands of operative procedures on hundreds of transfeminine patients. This book is not a guide for other doctors on facial feminization surgery.

We hope the information in this book will answer your questions and clarify the facial feminization process. It is a process that is sure to demand your patience and take up a good deal of your resources and time.

We want you to realize that even without gender reassignment surgery, you can achieve a more feminine face. Our past patients are a testament to the positive effect of these surgeries. They are doing exceedingly well, and some are even among the most beautiful women in the world!

Passing the Torch to Dr. Jordan Deschamps-Braly

When I wrote the first edition of this book, it was my intention to find a surgeon to take over and continue my life's work. Over the succeeding years, I struggled to find the right surgeon. Surgeons with the right training in the three necessary specialties—plastic surgery, craniofacial surgery, and orthognathic (jaw) surgery—are very rare.

It is even more unusual to find a surgeon with the right expertise who also has an interest in performing this type of work. Although several surgeons came to San Francisco to visit my practice, none were the right candidate.

Then, in 2014, I learned that a young craniofacial surgeon trained by Dr. Arlen Denny, an expert in that field, had recently begun practicing in San Francisco. That young surgeon was Dr. Jordan Deschamps-Braly. He had previously trained in all three of the essential specialties required for safe and effective facial feminization surgery. I was also personally acquainted with each of the four superb surgeons with whom he had trained. As Dr. Deschamps-Braly and I began to go to the operating room together, it was quickly apparent that he was, in fact, exactly the right surgeon to continue my life's work.

For nearly two years before my complete retirement, I continued to work in the operating room as Dr. Deschamps-Braly's assistant. From our first trip to the operating room, it was obvious that Dr. Deschamps-Braly's surgical planning, skills, organization, and execution are exceptional.

More importantly, over time, he has modified and improved several of the procedures we first used. As a result, the typical time in the operating room has been reduced for our patients while still providing excellent aesthetic results. His rate of complications is very low and similar to my personal experience over the previous thirty years.

It has been my pleasure to observe the skill, passion, and innovation that Dr. Deschamps-Braly has brought to the field of facial feminization surgery.

Now, in full retirement, the results I continue to observe in my periodic interactions with Dr. Deschamps-Braly's patients have easily exceeded my highest expectations. He is a worthy successor who will continue to care for my patients, and further this still very new field of surgery.

—DOUGLAS K. OUSTERHOUT, M.D., D.D.S.

1

Facial Feminization Surgery:
An Overview

LOOKING FEMININE IS CRUCIAL FOR
you. After all, first impressions are often based
only on your face. Others' perceptions of who
you are can also be shaped by your looks. So,
if you are, a transgender individual, nothing is
more important than having a face and body
that match how you feel. *Facial feminization
surgery (FFS)* can help you achieve a female
appearance. It helps you look like the person
you have always been on the inside.

Why Facial Feminization?

There is only one reason to feminize your
face: You want to appear female. You want to
be seen and thought of as being feminine in
every way. If you do not look the part, others
will identify you and speak to you as if you are
a man. The more feminine your face appears,
the more relaxed you become because you are
consistently identified as a woman.

Still, we have seen new developments in gender identification in contemporary times. Most
patients seeking feminization surgery are truly
"binary" and completely conform to the opposite

gender and use traditional he/she pronouns. Yet,
an increasing number do not identify with either
gender (gender nonconforming or nonbinary),
and use "they/them" pronouns.

These patients also seek facial surgery. Their
goal is to appear less like their birth-assigned
sex. So, facial feminization surgery may be more
appropriately called *gender neutralization surgery.*

There are many things to consider when
deciding whether to move forward with facial
feminization because it entails undergoing
serious surgery. For starters, how does facial
feminization fit in with *gender confirmation
surgery of the genitals* or *chest (GCS),* also
known as *gender reassignment surgery (GRS)*? If
you choose both, which should come first? And,
after you have decided to feminize your face,
which features should your surgeon target and
in what order?

By the time you finish this book, you should
be able to make informed choices about these
and other FFS matters. But first, let's look at

MALE

FEMALE

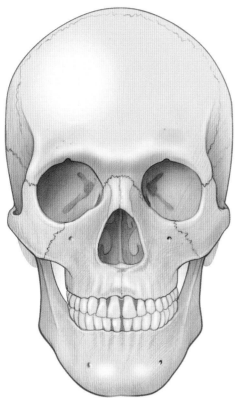

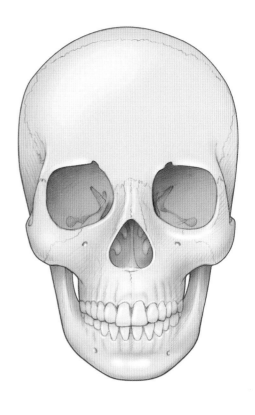

The male skull is more rectangular and has a vertically longer chin and a wider, fuller jaw.

The female skull is more oval and has a vertically shorter, more pointed chin.

the facial differences between the genders that make this surgery necessary.

Differences in Male and Female Facial Structures

Anthropologists and artists alike, have long appreciated the basic differences between the skulls of men and women. Fueled by the male hormone testosterone in puberty, masculine facial features are more prominent than feminine features. Men have vertically longer and less pointed chins with less tapered jaws than women. Male noses are also larger than those of females. Men have what we call *bossing,* a rounded prominence of the lower forehead behind the brows.

It extends from the mid-forehead laterally to the outside of the bony eye sockets. A woman's forehead, on the other hand, is continually convex, and curves outward with less forward projection than a man's forehead.

As you read this book, you will learn just how feminization surgery can erase each of these differences. A surgeon with expertise in FFS can significantly reduce and contour the skeletal structures underneath key facial features. That surgeon can turn the larger size, angles, and proportions found in men's faces into the smaller size, angles, and proportions found in women.

MALE

FEMALE

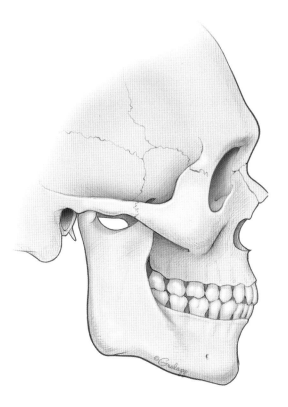

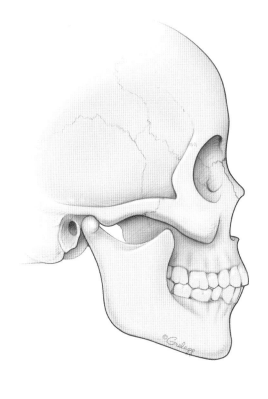

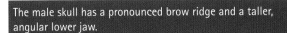

The male skull has a pronounced brow ridge and a taller, angular lower jaw.

The female skull has a more rounded smooth forehead that does not project over the eyes and a shorter, tapered lower jaw.

Although facial feminization can help you be perceived as a woman, you may wonder how important it is in comparison to gender confirmation surgery of the genitals or chest. This may be especially true if the cost of having both surgeries does not fit into your budget. Let's take a closer look at the two options. It may help you weigh your choices.

Demographics of Facial Feminization Patients

The age distribution of people who come to us for facial feminization is changing. A decade ago, our patients were typically middle-aged individuals, with an average age between forty-four and fifty-eight. (Our two oldest patients were age seventy-one and seventy-four—evidence that it is never too late if you are healthy.)

These patients are people who have staved off their feminine feelings for years by getting married, having children, and even entering male-dominated fields such as athletics, police, and the military. Eventually, however, they find the emotional forces within themselves too great to ignore and they yield to them, seeking the female world.

More recently, we see a shift toward younger people (often in their twenties and thirties) who have decided to live as females, and sometimes seek facial feminization.

Another group includes those individuals who have previously passed as females. They could pass very well as females in their twenties and thirties, but as they age, they have found that their faces become more masculine. So, they undergo facial feminization.

Today, an increasing number of young people in their teens or even earlier are aware that they are transgender individuals. But that does not mean they are ready for FFS. The male skull may not be fully developed until age eighteen, and, in some cases, even later. So, it is not wise to have these procedures until your plastic surgeon is confident that your facial growth is complete. Otherwise, you risk needing further surgery later in life.

How do you know when you have stopped developing? The best way to tell is with radiographs of the growth plates of the wrist. Closure of the growth plates tends to indicate that growth has ceased. Age is generally also a good predictor. Chances are, that if you are not getting any taller by your late teens, your facial skeleton will not change much, even if you are not fully biologically mature.

The youngest patient either of us has ever feminized was seventeen years old, and obviously it was performed only with parental consent and encouragement. Several individuals were age eighteen or nineteen when we completed their surgeries. In all those cases, we were confident that the facial bone structure and skull were ready enough, so that we would not have to repeat the surgeries.

FFS vs. "Top" or "Bottom" Surgery

Many individuals believe that *gender confirmation surgery* of the genitals or chest are the primary steps for transitioning to female. Certainly, surgically modifying male genitalia into female genitalia is an obvious and significant alteration for someone who wants to change gender. Having worked for more than three decades in this arena, our sense is that more transgender individuals select bottom surgery and top surgery over FFS than the reverse. They have decided, for financial or personal reasons, that undergoing gender confirmation surgery of the genitals or chest is more desirable than having a feminine face. For them, this surgery is indeed a giant step forward.

There are few validated statistics on the number of people who undergo bottom surgery, top surgery, and FFS worldwide. Also, the statistics that exist are likely inaccurate because they rely on self-reporting by patients and individual doctors. Yet, trends are changing. We see an increasing number of patients who feel that "socially" transitioning is impossible without feminizing the face. For those individuals, FFS is infinitely more important to their quality of life than is the reassignment of genitalia.

Our thinking is that being regarded as a female is the most important step in transitioning. Yes, even more important than vaginoplasty. In the past, there have been dissenters who argue against facial feminization (for starters, some see it as an expensive, misdirected act), but we strongly disagree. In addition, there is a strong correlation between facial feminization surgery and positive psychological outcomes.

Changing your masculine features to reflect the smaller angles and proportions of a female

FEMALE   **MALE**

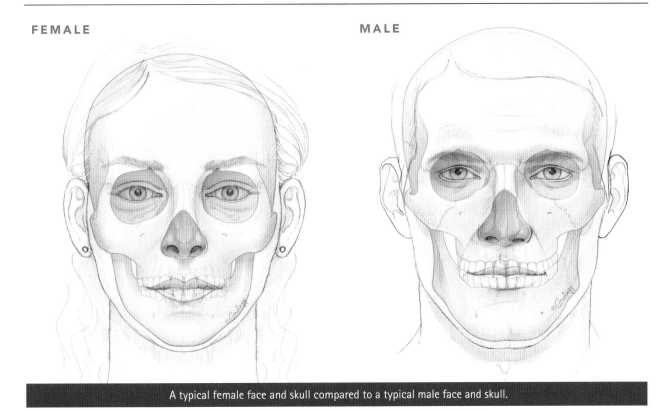

A typical female face and skull compared to a typical male face and skull.

face has many positive benefits. First, it eliminates or markedly reduces any immediate visually detectable remnant of masculinity. Unfortunately, even after undergoing GCS, transgender individuals still retain their male facial features, making it difficult for them to assimilate into society as women. If you choose to have genital surgery, facial feminization can pave the way. Finally, it helps you feel more like a female when you walk down the street. We have met many patients who found great satisfaction in transforming their faces, whether or not they underwent top surgery or bottom surgery.

Choosing FFS Alone

Just as some individuals are adamant about having top or bottom surgery, either with or without FFS, others primarily want to look feminine. They don't feel the need to change their

genitalia to be socially accepted. Or perhaps they wish to remain in the masculine world, at least part of the time, but still want to "pass" in the feminine world. Several of our patients over the years have continued to work and be regarded as men by day and dressed as women at night without any problems.

They have managed well because males can have a feminine face and still be accepted. By contrast, females may have difficulty with gender identification if they appear too masculine. These individuals move comfortably between the two worlds, functioning as men when dressed as a male, and as women when dressed as a female. If you desire this living arrangement, a feminized face should not be a problem for you in the male world.

Undergoing Facial Feminization Surgery

Facial feminization requires aggressive facial and bone surgeries designed to reshape the masculine areas of your skull. These procedures contour the forehead, eye sockets, nose, jaw, and chin, while reducing the Adam's apple, lips, and pattern of hair growth. With this collection of procedures, your surgeon can provide you with a look and profile that befits a woman.

Patients often ask us why a facelift will not garner the same positive results as FFS. We remind them that just as you can't change the shape of a house with a coat of paint, you can't feminize the skull by only lifting the skin. In other words, you must address the underlying foundation, in this case, the bony structures, to affect the outside contours. Even though a facelift may be a desirable add-on, altering the skeleton is the only way to change a patient's appearance from distinctly male to distinctly female.

As you will learn, feminizing some facial areas is more important than feminizing others. Still, information on all the procedures we do—including results, recovery, and potential complications—are detailed in this book.

Although modifying every area of the face can be key to a feminine appearance, people do not always need to change everything. In fact, facial feminization is a very individualized process. Each person has a unique face and, more importantly, a unique bony structure underlying that face. So, what a surgeon does for one transgender individual may be totally different for another transgender patient. As was mentioned earlier, there are some male characteristics that need to be eliminated or refined for any transgender individual to pass as feminine. Yet, each change should be targeted to that person's face. There are no cookie-cutter procedures in this process!

Sequence of FFS Procedures

After you have decided on FFS, the next choice you will make concerns the timing of your procedures. Will they occur before or after GRS/GCS, if you are having both? Will you have all your facial feminization surgeries in one trip to the operating room or in separate surgeries?

Among our transfeminine patients who undergo both gender reassignment and facial feminization, more individuals than not, seem to want FFS first. Yet, although we have treated a very large number of patients, they are only a portion of the larger transgender community. For that reason, we are not certain our observation remains valid in the larger transgender population. To this day, there are no national statistics on FFS surgeries. There is most likely little hope that accurate statistics can be generated because of the requirement for self-reporting by patients. And surveying surgical specialists about their work may also be of limited value due to their reluctance to disclose their practice profiles.

We have treated some patients who had gender confirmation procedures ten to twenty-five years ago, and now want a more feminine look. They may have presented easily as women in their twenties and thirties, but as they enter their forties, they want a more feminine look. Also, very little was known about facial feminization three decades ago, so they had no choice in the initial procedures available.

After you have made your decision about undergoing FFS, it is usually advantageous to complete all the operations at one time because of cost and recovery time; however, it is not a necessity.

Five percent of patients start out with only a reduction of their thyroid cartilage or Adam's apple, one of the most prominent masculine characteristics. The Adam's apple is a dead give-away to your status. Some patients choose to divide the procedures into two sessions, usually for monetary, job, family, or relationship reasons. We usually insist on combining certain procedures, specifically the forehead and the nose, or, alternatively, the chin and the jaw. They must be feminized together for reasons that we explain in subsequent chapters.

Those individuals who want to separate their feminization surgeries often ask us which area—the upper or lower face—should be addressed first. We usually suggest beginning with the most masculine features. If they are of equal concern in our eyes, we leave it up to our patients.

Recovery and Follow-up Care

Facial feminization may be elective surgery, but it is surgery all the same. You will look worse before you look better. Expect to be swollen, and to some extent bruised. In the first edition of this book, opioid painkillers were discussed as a normal part of the expected recovery process. However, that is no longer true.

In 2013, we developed a new, enhanced recovery protocol based mostly on anti-inflammatory medications. This protocol has allowed almost all of our patients to avoid all opioid-based pain medication. We also use other peer-reviewed techniques that reduce inflammation and speed healing. Our patients now rarely complain of postsurgical pain that exceeds a level of "2" or "3" on a 10-point pain scale.

Avoiding opioid narcotics after surgery significantly improves your recovery and prevents any risk of addiction. It also dramatically reduces swelling after surgery. We insist that

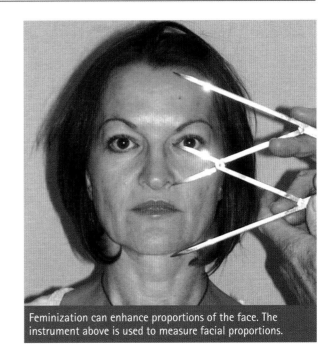

Feminization can enhance proportions of the face. The instrument above is used to measure facial proportions.

our patients begin walking shortly after surgery because it helps clear the anesthetics from the system and reduces swelling. However, you should not jog or do any vigorous activity for several weeks after surgery. You'll also have to adjust your diet if your mouth needs to heal. If you are one of the rare patients who needs medications for pain, they will be prescribed for you.

It will take a year or more before you see the complete results of your surgery. Generally, we say it takes two or three weeks to be presentable in public. Patients continue to see considerable improvement for two to three months afterward. In six to eight weeks, you will be able to return to your usual activities, sporting a fresh, feminized face. However, improvement continues for up to eighteen months in some cases.

Returning to Work

Returning to work is a very important issue for most people. If our patients can work from a computer at home, they can go back to work as soon as they feel up to it. You might start with a work schedule of just a few hours per day. For unknown and curious reasons, many of our patients are software engineers. These patients are not just from the San Francisco Bay area, but from around the globe. Some of these patients find they can even work the day after surgery.

If you must go to a workplace and mingle with other people, however, you may want to wait two to three weeks. Depending on your age, it may take you this much time to easily return to your workplace. If you do heavy labor, you should probably plan on taking a month off. Still, the question of when to return to work is more of a social issue than a practical one. If coworkers or social acquaintances are aware that surgery is being done, then an abbreviated absence is all that is necessary because no one at work will be surprised by bruising and swelling that naturally go along with surgery. When significant secrecy surrounds the surgery process, however, then a longer time away from public view is helpful.

What will you look like afterward? Our primary objective, no matter which facial feminization procedures you undergo, is that you can pass easily as a female. What constitutes "passing"? It is being able to function in the world as a female without question. It is answering the door on an early Saturday morning without your lipstick, makeup, or usual hairdo, and hearing the visitor say, "I am very sorry to bother you, ma'am."

Will You Look Beautiful after Surgery?

Beauty is the one thing we cannot promise from facial feminization. Beauty is a very elusive concept, difficult to describe and even harder to deliver. Plastic surgeons have wrestled with the notion of beauty ever since they began resculpting faces. However, no one has yet come up with the ultimate "ah-ha-this-is-it" objective

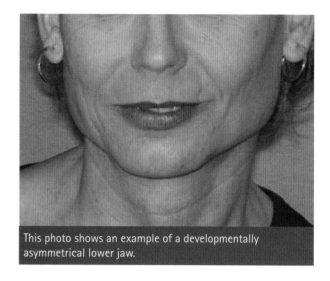

This photo shows an example of a developmentally asymmetrical lower jaw.

definition. Beauty is in the eye of the beholder, after all.

Yet, some have tried to characterize beauty. Scientists, for instance, have used all sorts of devices to define a beautiful face. A colleague tried averaging the cephalograms—radiographic images of the craniofacial skeleton—of beauty queens or images of the craniofacial area to produce the most perfect facial skeleton. Did it work? Not particularly well.

We all have our own perceptions of handsome or pretty. If ten men were asked to pick the most beautiful among 100 attractive women, probably none would make the same choice.

Our perceptions of beauty are defined by ethnicity and the experiences of everyday life. Our society has a bias toward European beauty standards, but each racial and ethnic group is uniquely beautiful.

The media, peer pressure, and sexual preferences influence what we find attractive. Cultural norms also affect what we do to make ourselves appealing, especially to the opposite sex. From haute couture to hairstyles, we choose based on our own personalities and what looks good on us. Often, these choices are dictated by complexions, bone structures, and even facial fat.

Beauty Is Still Important to Feminization

Not surprisingly, beauty is such an important concept that patients naturally want a great aesthetic result from facial feminization. Everyone hopes to look their very best. For the surgeon, paying attention to that goal is essential at each step of the operation—from evaluating the patient to planning and executing the surgery. Careful follow-up during postoperative recovery is also needed to attain the best results.

Achieving the most pleasing aesthetic effects in facial feminization requires surgical skill, experience, and even artistry.

As we reconstruct a patient's face, surgeons must keep both mathematical and artistic concepts in mind. Primarily these are *proportion*, or the relationship between individual features and the whole face, and *symmetry*, whether there are similarities between corresponding sides of the face.

Proportion Is a Key Guideline

Facial proportion is perhaps the single most important consideration in producing a beautiful result. Some people suggest that all beauty is a matter of proportion, expressed by an ancient mathematical concept called the *Golden Mean.* The Golden Mean is a mathematical formula that quantifies the proportional relationship between the whole and its parts. Whether in nature, architecture, art, or anatomy, the most beautiful examples adhere to the Golden Mean. That includes the faces of women. In fact, attractive women almost always express this constant ratio.

Feminization can markedly improve the proportions of a transfeminine individual. How so?

By reducing the height of several facial areas, a surgeon can alter the dimensions and proportions dramatically to fit a smaller feminine face.

When the scalp and hairline are advanced, for instance, forehead height is reduced. When the chin is shortened, the entire length of the face is decreased. Similarly, when the length and width of the nose and the height of the upper lip is diminished, the face will appear more feminine.

Must every transgender face be made vertically shorter? Not necessarily, even though this is usually what's needed. Whether your features need to be shortened or lengthened, your surgeon's goal must be to establish correct proportions in your finished face.

Symmetry in Facial Features

The idea that perfect symmetry is the key to beauty is a popular misconception. If one looks at the faces of public figures, who are considered beautiful, most will exhibit significant asymmetry. In fact, the face of every individual is asymmetrical to some extent.

Perfect symmetry is actually quite disturbing to the eye. Having perfect symmetry makes the face appear like two identical right- or left-sided mirrored images. In fact, a 2017 review study in the *Aesthetic Surgery Journal* provided strong scientific support for the idea that too much asymmetry is not attractive. Furthermore, too much symmetry will appear unsightly.

Symmetry can be evaluated in several ways:

- *by looking closely at an individual*
- *by looking down on his or her face from above*
- *by measuring the distances from the midline of the face at various points*
- *by using a specialized mirror to allow patients to see more clearly the asymmetries of their own face*

If your countenance is extremely asymmetrical, some areas of your face and skull can be corrected, although others may be difficult or even impossible to alter. Fortunately, the contouring steps taken during facial feminization can markedly improve lower facial asymmetries. By tapering the lower jaw and realigning the chin, your surgeon can improve the balance in your lower face.

The *facial profile*—or the view of the face from the side—is also an important aspect of any beautiful face. A stunning profile has a significant impact on one's appearance. To our minds, a beautiful profile is one in which all the features fit together. Is there one perfect example? No. Profiles vary tremendously, yet the most beautiful profiles exhibit an aesthetically pleasing relationship between the parts. The features must be in harmony. Extreme profiles may show "character," but they are rarely beautiful.

Yet even with attention to proportion, symmetry, profile, and other factors (such as skin color and texture, teeth, and hair), no surgeon can guarantee a beautiful result. In fact, the bottom-line question for you is, "Are you willing to go through facial feminization if you end up looking like a woman, but not a beautiful woman?" If the answer is no, FFS is not for you. If the answer is yes, however, rest assured. By focusing on aesthetics and being technically skilled, your surgeon should be able to deliver a positive result. And yes, some of our patients even meet that elusive definition of "beautiful."

> *FFS really was an investment, because it allowed me to sustain my career, retire early, and do stuff I wanted to do. I haven't felt a need to have anything done since then, and the surgery I had over twenty years ago still serves me well today.*

Living with a Feminine Face: You Will Adapt Quickly

We have found that our patients acclimate to their new faces so swiftly that after the dressings come off, they seem to forget what they looked like previously. It is amazing that the mind is able to make that shift in perception. However, sometimes the mind plays tricks on us. On occasion a patient may say, "I don't look any different than I did before surgery." Yet, when we review their preoperative photographs, they can appreciate the marked transformation that has taken place. They see a resemblance to the past, but the structures of the face, such as the forehead, nose, and chin, are definitely more feminine.

You may have the same experience as many others we have treated. You will likely resemble your mother when she was younger or your sister as she is today. Even if you looked more like your father before the procedures, you will look distinctly feminine. As your healing progresses after surgery, your face will also appear increasingly feminine. With time (usually within a few months post-surgery), you'll move even further away from your male face. Instead, you'll have a feminine face that you will appreciate.

Reactions from Others

Patients often ask us what they can expect from friends and family, and how they should handle others' initial responses after surgery. People who see you on a regular basis, and even know that you are having facial feminization, will no doubt recognize you. They might even say they don't see a difference. We have recommended keeping a preoperative picture handy, so you can show them how surgery made a considerable difference in your appearance. After they make the comparison, chances are they will say, "Wow, what a difference!"

Old friends, like the close friends you knew from high school or the classmates you caroused with in college, might not recognize you at all, however. Your best pal may even pass you at a class reunion or ignore you at the next alumni function, unaware of who you are. You may need to break the ice or make the connection. Take your lead from how much this person seems to know and decide beforehand what you want to share.

One last word on the reactions of others. Some of our patients tell us that people still react to them as male even after surgery. *Our advice:* Think about whether you are being needlessly self-conscious. If anyone stares at you after facial surgery, it is likely because you look very attractive. Chances are, that this person is admiring you and nothing else.

We have encountered another interesting issue that occurs even after the most successful surgeries. A patient may say she is uniformly gender-identified correctly in public but cannot escape the image of her former self in the mirror. This is rare, yet it does come up from time to time. The solution in this scenario is rarely to undergo more surgery. Often, the solution is simply time for further healing. Also, if you have a psychotherapist, perhaps your therapist can help you work through these difficulties.

A surprisingly large percentage of our patients tend to be tall, even for people assigned male at birth. They sometimes worry that their physical height will cause them to be perceived as male, even after their FFS surgery. Some of our patients who are tall report that they do

get attention when they are in public. They have come to appreciate this attention, however, because it occurs only because they appear to be strikingly beautiful females. One caveat, however: Facial feminization does not alter your mannerisms or the pitch of your voice. So, if you think there is lingering suspicion about your gender, you might want to work on both.

A Final Note

In recent years, there have been significant improvements in the social recognition and acceptance of transgender people. More trans adolescents are taking female hormones to make their secondary male sex characteristics less overt. If this trend continues, facial feminization surgery will still be necessary, but the surgeries may be less comprehensive while achieving even more beautiful results. Injected hormones don't have the same effect on the facial skeleton as they do on the rest of the body, yet they do stimulate changes in hair distribution and hairline height.

Even if you are taking hormones, FFS can be extremely beneficial in helping you pass as a female and blend comfortably with the rest of society. Yes, you can live your life as a woman without facial feminization procedures. In fact, you may function very well. But you run the very real risk that your masculine features will get in the way of being socially accepted as a female.

Facial feminization can help match your exterior appearance to the way you feel on the inside. Many of our patients make comments such as: "I no longer fear looking at my face in the mirror when I get out of bed each morning." Instead, the vision of one's face glimpsed in a mirror is a source of self-confidence and joy.

2

Preparing for
Facial Feminization Surgery

NO SURGERY, including facial feminization surgery, should be undertaken lightly. As with gender confirmation surgery, a decision to have facial feminization surgery requires a good deal of soul-searching and planning. Reshaping the bones of your face and skull is a serious undertaking. It requires preparation, knowledge, and attention to detail. It may take time and effort to find a surgeon who has developed the right skills and can understand all the nuances of the procedures covered in this book. What should you do to prepare yourself for the procedure? Our goal is to provide you with the information you need to make the right decisions—for you!

Choosing a Plastic Surgeon

Whenever you have surgery, it's best to select a physician who is both highly trained and experienced. This is particularly important when the operation involves remodeling the bony structures of your face. The formal training that enables a surgeon to do this surgery safely requires training in three specialties: plastic surgery, maxillofacial surgery, and craniofacial surgery. A surgeon with just one or two out of these three qualifications should not be acceptable.

Unfortunately, some surgeons who present themselves as qualified to do these surgeries, are not even properly trained or qualified in any single one of those three essential surgical specialties. Whatever reconstructive or cosmetic surgical procedure you are seeking, you must do your homework to find the right surgeon.

After reading this book, you should have a better idea of what is important, and you will be able to ask a potential plastic surgeon much better questions. (For detailed information about how to evaluate surgeons' training, skills, and experience, see Appendix A.)

Be Cautious about Information from the Internet

Should you use the internet to check out your surgeon? Yes, but with caution. The internet puts many resources and information about doctors at your fingertips. You can scope out the websites of individual surgeons and their

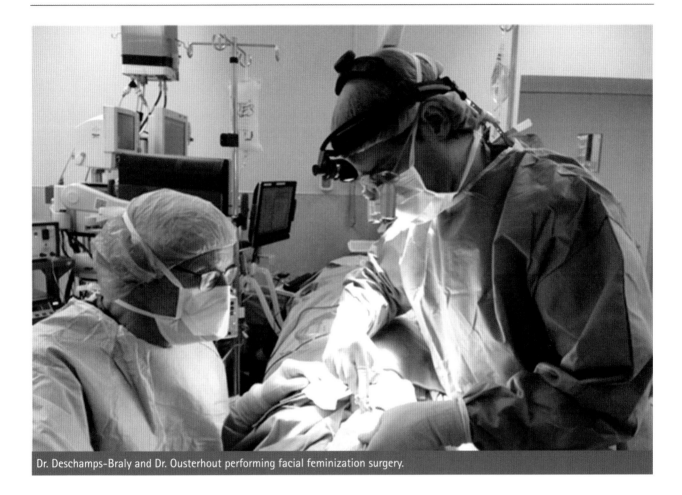

Dr. Deschamps-Braly and Dr. Ousterhout performing facial feminization surgery.

professional credentials. You can also read what other patients have written about their surgeons through various web pages and message boards.

Yet, you need to conduct internet searches wisely. Although surfing the web is generally a good idea, be wary about the content. There is a lot of misleading information on the internet about facial feminization—from the recovery stories (the postoperative pain, scars, and numbness) to the overall results.

In the past, the misinformation seemed to have come from individuals who had never had these surgeries. Yet, they wanted to discourage others from undergoing FFS. One wonders about their motives.

However, another phenomenon is now occurring on the internet. There has been a significant increase in social media postings, essentially influencers, intending to promote various surgeons' practices.

High-quality information and patient reports about their experiences with an FFS surgeon can be very helpful. But also consider that some individuals' emotional investment in the results of their surgeries can shade their descriptions. Often, patients post extended descriptions about their surgeries—but their photos show significant shortcomings in the results achieved. In such postings, there is often little or no evidence of any honest or constructive feedback.

If you have reliable information, you can ably evaluate any false reports about FFS that you encounter. By reading this book, you will be in a better position to weigh derogatory comments or incorrect information on the internet. Likewise, you will be able to more accurately appreciate the merits of truly excellent results when they are presented.

One significant and growing problem is that physicians who do not know how to do certain procedures will say that FFS is experimental, painful, or causes many complications. Still, other physicians, with limited training and abilities, will try to retain a patient's interest in their services by suggesting that FFS is unnecessary. Yet, patients may need these procedures if they want a fully feminine face.

Make sure you get balanced viewpoints in the information you read. If you obtain information from others during social interactions, weigh it carefully. In every case, do a gut check on your emotions and consider the source. Then proceed with your educated and rational evaluation.

Be Skeptical about Before and After Pictures on Internet Forums

This caution arises out of a growing problem. Much too often, we have had patients bring to their consultations before and after pictures of another patient whose procedure was performed by another surgeon, and ask if such results are realistic or possible. This seems to happen more often with foreign surgery centers and foreign surgeons, but it is also a growing problem in the United States and Canada. In a few cases from outside the United States, the before and after photos do not even show the same individual, or if they do show the same individual, then the pictures

have been skillfully edited. The signs of such digital editing can be subtle, such as not scaling the pictures properly, so that the postoperative photo appears smaller than the preoperative photo. Giveaway features in those photographs are changes in facial features that cannot be accomplished by surgery.

Be Skeptical about Before and After Pictures on Surgeons' Websites

Our office has established a firm policy of not posting patient pictures online. At first, we received criticism by patients who wanted to see the surgical results of FFS without coming in for a consultation. But, as we anticipated, within less than a year, patients began to genuinely appreciate this policy. After all, it was adopted due to ethical concerns and to protect the privacy of patients. Even patients who have given their permission for their photos to be used may later regret this decision, due to changes in personal circumstances. However, the internet is forever.

Keep in mind that the use of patient before and after photos on the internet has now been seriously corrupted by some surgeons. They often make skillful use of pictures with heavy concealing makeup, favorable lighting, or digital image manipulation.

As board-certified plastic surgeons in the United States, we are prohibited by our written ethical standards from publishing or using pictures that are misleading to the public or prospective patients.

Question. Are you absolutely sure who will physically perform your surgery? It is not always who you think it will be. In some practices, residents in training programs may perform portions of your surgery, rather than the surgeon you see for consultation.

How Pictures Should Be Presented

In our practice, we keep a large volume of before and after photos in our office. We show these photos during face-to-face consultations; the photos frequently bring up discussions about the results that can be realistically achieved, given your desires and facial features. The photos include young patients, those who are more mature, and patients of different races. All our office photos are taken under identical lighting conditions with neutral backgrounds and similar hair arrangement.

There is absolutely no digital editing or manipulation of the images. In some instances, patients returning for checkups weeks or months after surgery will be photographed in our office as they now appear in their daily lives. However, the circumstances will always be obvious or clearly identified. We are grateful to our many patients who have given us permission to use their pictures in our private office setting, for our professional presentations, medical publications, and in this book.

When looking at photos of former patients during a consultation with a surgeon, you may also want to ask if these patients are willing to discuss their facial feminization surgery. Keep in mind that the availability of such former patients for conversations changes from month to month. Decisions by former patients to continue to communicate (or not) with other patients in transition are extremely personal decisions and we respect their privacy.

Although your doctor cannot legally give out individual names, some will ask a consenting former patient to contact you. In that case, it is up to you to ask detailed questions. If the two of you are comfortable, you can exchange names. You might even want to meet face to face.

Is Surgery Abroad a Bad Option?

As a U.S. or Canadian resident, should you go abroad for FFS? A number of individuals research having surgery abroad as a way of saving money. You can find surgeons who advertise themselves as FFS surgeons in Asia, Latin or South America, and Europe. Just because you could go there and undergo the surgery does not mean it is a safe idea. *Medical tourism* (or global health care) is a growth industry that began several years ago and now includes many areas of medicine, including plastic surgery. The term reflects the rapidly growing number of people who are willing to travel across international borders to obtain elective health services, often at a savings they consider significant.

Yet, scientific and journalistic investigations into medical tourism have revealed that it is not always what it seems to be. There are potential downsides to medical tourism, especially for transfeminine individuals searching for ways to obtain facial feminization. If you undergo surgery this way, you will be outside the "safe harbor" of well-established modern Western medicine.

By leaving the United States or Canada, you lose the ability to use long-established, independent, third-party professional organizations who vet and certify the quality, training, and experience of surgeons and medical facilities. (See Appendix A for details.) In those circumstances, you cannot fully evaluate the qualifications of prospective surgeons. You also lose the ability to know how safe the facility is in which your surgery will be performed. At an absolute minimum, your ability to have family or friends assist you becomes limited; having family members travel with you creates, additional expenses.

Europeans have now established board-certification entities that are similar to those in the United States. (See Appendix A section on board certification.) As noted in Appendix A, however, there are few surgeons in Europe who are widely known for facial feminization surgery and have the necessary board certifications.

Occasionally, surgeons who do not have legitimate board certifications, make claims to have the training needed to perform FFS. They may even list their medical training history. Yet, on closer scrutiny, their purported board certifications are not legitimate, and/or the certifications come from organizations that are not widely accepted in the medical community. Sometimes, these "alternative" board certifications are referred to as "vanity" or "marketing" certifications.

You may ask: "Aren't all doctors trained and prepared in the same way?" The answer is simply "no." In structured curriculums such as those in the United States, Canada, the United Kingdom, Australia, and certain EU countries, the path to a medical practice is a well-defined and controlled process that involves many checks and balances. For example, in the United States, a surgeon must complete four years of college, three years of medical school, and at least five years of hands-on residency training.

Many doctors, including the two of us, choose to continue on with one or more specialty fellowships to expand our skills and knowledge. We both spent many years in excess of our plastic surgery training receiving additional experience in craniofacial surgery. Along the way, each surgeon must show competency through testing and experience to be licensed to practice in any state.

Surgical privileges at good United States and Canadian hospitals are generally limited to those surgeons who are board-certified in a recognized surgical field. Yet, such rigorous training and board certifications are not required in many foreign countries. In contrast, U.S. and Canadian hospitals, clinics, and other medical facilities must meet stringent standards to be accredited and licensed to deliver surgical services.

Unfortunately, other countries vary in their medical standards. Although you should always be concerned with any surgeon's credentials, as well as a medical facility's readiness to deliver safe care, it is particularly important in a nation where training and certifications are different and less stringently controlled than in the United States. Wherever you go, make sure you understand the training your surgeon has undergone in order to be completely competent to perform FFS.

If you are thinking of obtaining FFS surgery in a foreign country, here are a few questions you should ask:

- *Is the surgeon in a foreign country actually a properly trained and experienced plastic surgeon?*

- *Did the surgeon complete a plastic surgery residency?*

- *Did the surgeon finish a maxillofacial surgery fellowship?*

- *Did the surgeon complete a full craniofacial surgery fellowship?*

- *Can you verify the claims made about the surgeon's training?*

- *How does the surgeon approach the facial areas described in this book?*

- *Does the surgeon actually have experience in facial feminization surgery, or did the surgeon simply watch another surgeon do one case, and proclaim to be an expert?*

- *Does the surgeon allow student doctors to participate or do parts of the procedure?*

You need to know as much as possible about who is doing the work and where it is being done. Remember, this is your face.

Also, consider an important fact: The surgeon whose procedures do not result in at least an occasional complication, is the surgeon who does not operate. In other words, the best of surgeons will have at least one patient who experiences a complication. What happens if you are the patient who suffers that occasional postsurgical complication? If your original surgeon is professionally respected, it will be easier to find a local surgeon who can deal with any complication that arises.

However, if your original surgeon was not fully trained and qualified, then when you return home your local surgeon may be far less enthusiastic about dealing with a complication. Fixing another surgeon's mistakes is not always possible and can take considerable time.

A growing number of patients routinely come to us after other surgeons have failed to give them a pleasing aesthetic result. Examples include the following:

- *The forehead wasn't reduced properly.*
- *The nose doesn't look as feminine as it should.*
- *The chin is now asymmetrical.*
- *Too little was removed from the lower jaw.*
- *The chin was not adequately shortened.*
- *In some cases, the original surgery left the patient with only a whisper of a voice.*

In 2008, approximately 8 percent of Dr. Ousterhout's patients were "revisions" from other surgeons. Currently, the proportion of our office consultations and surgeries for patients seeking revisions due to unsatisfactory results by other surgeons continues to increase. As of 2019, approximately 15 percent of our patients who come in for consultations are seeking revisions to correct the outcome of surgeries performed elsewhere. Most often, we can address the needs of these patients. Unfortunately, in some cases, revisions may not be possible or the risks outweigh the possible benefits.

Usually, these adverse outcomes are the results of surgeries performed by inexperienced, foreign practitioners. In some cases, these poor outcomes result from surgeries in the United States. For example, we recently examined a younger patient who believed her forehead had been unfavorably altered. Her first surgeon is a prominent surgeon in another city. However, the patient was unhappy because the results were not consistent with the results of other women who underwent the same forehead surgery. When we reviewed her X-rays, it was clear that the surgery she had paid for and which was documented in her medical records—called a *Type III forehead surgery*—had never been performed.

Yes, she had the surgical scar from the earlier surgery, but the remodeling of the frontal sinus cavity that is an important part of this surgery, had never been done. We subsequently performed a Type III forehead procedure, and the patient ended up with results that should have been achieved with her first surgery.

The unfortunate reality for these patients is that there is a cost to correcting another doctor's complications and outright mistakes. A revision of another surgeon's complications or mistakes is often difficult. It takes longer than a first-time effort. Very often, a patient expects the ideal result that she did not get the first

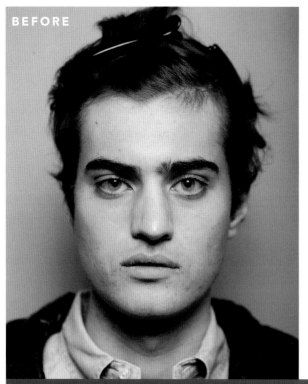
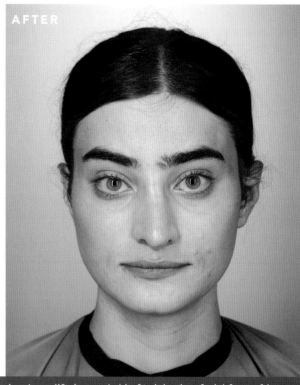

FFS procedures included: scalp advancement, Type III forehead contouring, brow lift, jaw and chin feminization, facial fat grafting, thyroid cartilage reduction, rhinoplasty, and septoplasty to reshape bone and cartilage structures between the nostrils.

time. Yet, sometimes the problem cannot be corrected—it can only be improved.

If you are traveling outside the country for health care, you may have no medical or legal recourse should something go very wrong. We have seen the CT scans and surgical outcomes of some patients who have had surgery outside the United States. The X-ray and photographic documentation of those surgeries is distressing to any well-trained surgeon. The results were also a nightmare for the patients.

Although insurance coverage for FFS is usually not available, parts of the surgery may be covered in the United States if there is an extenuating health reason. Yet, if you go abroad for your surgery, the procedures will almost certainly not be covered under any circumstances. In recent years, some insurance companies have begun to provide coverage, but often that is only through "in-network" surgeons. Rarely do those surgeons have the full range of training and experience required to properly and safely perform these surgeries. It is encouraging that, recently, some of the more prominent employers in the United States have begun supporting their employees with robust coverage for these surgeries.

If you honestly believe your best option is to leave the country, then please do some extra homework. Much is being written these days about the pluses and minuses of medical tourism. Make sure you talk to someone who has not only experienced facial feminization outside the country, but who also had problems with some aspect of the process. You can find them online.

You need to know what can go awry by taking your surgery out of the United States.

One caution: There appear to be representatives of some FFS surgery facilities who "bully" or intimidate anyone who expresses dissatisfaction online with their foreign surgery experience. Some personal accounts of FFS surgery—either positive or negative—that are posted online are simply unreliable.

Also, be wary of information that you obtain from an extended email message chain whose title line resembles the following, "My surgery with [name of surgeon] in April of this year in [city, name of country]."

Some of these types of messages are legitimate, but others are usually targeted advertising. Often, they are written by a patient who has obtained special discounts or free treatments from a surgeon with a heavily promoted practice.

Some message boards also refuse to allow almost any factual reports of adverse experiences with any surgeon. Moderators of FFS surgery forums are right to prohibit open "bashing" of surgeons. They have a difficult job in striking the right balance between allowing constructive criticism and avoiding angry surgeon bashing. Such surgeon-bashing may be based on erroneous information or misunderstanding of the surgeries and associated complications. On the other hand, constructive information, even if it is adverse, is useful for prospective patients.

Important: The majority of the poor FFS outcomes done through medical tourism appear to us to be a result of the patient's limited financial resources coupled with the natural impulse

> *Do not be surprised if your surgeon asks questions about when you first considered your transition. It is not an attempt to invade your privacy. Rather, it is the obligation of any surgeon to verify that you are ready for transformational surgery like FFS.*

to quickly move forward with a transition. That combination of circumstances is manifested in the patient's decision to seek out and obtain complex facial surgery from the least expensive surgeon, often in a medical tourism location.

If you fit that description, consider that it is usually better to be more patient and make sure your surgery is performed properly the first time.

Your Consultations

You and your surgeon must accomplish many things during your initial office visits to determine your physical and emotional readiness for facial feminization. Because this is very aggressive skeletal surgery, no matter which procedures you undergo, you will want to know everything that is in store for you both pre- and postoperatively. Your doctor also has to find out if you are physically and emotionally ready and able to undergo these surgeries. Your doctor will make great efforts to see that you are in good physical health and that any medical conditions you have, are clearly under control.

Goals Are Important

During our initial consultation with patients, we address many issues, beginning with the reasons they want to have surgery and what they hope to achieve. Most importantly, every individual is asked a set of standard questions for which there are no right or wrong answers. The responses, however, are important in guiding our recommendations:

- *Are you on, or will you soon be starting, hormonal replacement therapy?*

- *Have you had, or will you have gender confirmation surgery of the genitals and chest? It is important to know this because sometimes placement of catheters during surgery can be complicated by a former genital surgery.*

- *What do you expect to look like after your facial feminization surgery?*

- *Will you undergo the surgery if there are no guarantees that you will be beautiful after healing is complete?*

- *How do you think the surgery is going to affect your life?*

We also want to know whether you have a therapist. However, we do not require a counselor's recommendation or letter approving FFS before proceeding with the surgeries. For FFS procedures, we do not ask our patients to undergo the real-life experience and test required prior to gender confirmation surgery of the genitals and chest (GRS/GCS). However, in our many years of performing facial feminization, we have very rarely operated on anyone who, in retrospect, was not ready for surgery. And yes, each of us has denied surgery to more than a few patients.

We and our patients recognize that undergoing facial feminization surgery takes a certain amount of maturity—first to submit to one or more major surgeries, second to accept a dramatic change in your facial appearance, and third, to really want to look feminine. Yes, it is true that you can be re-masculinized if you have a change of heart after your procedures. Yet, neither of us plastic surgeons have ever had to do this, not even once.

In fact, as far as we know, none of our patients have changed their minds about facial feminization. Not one has insisted on reversing the surgery, even though two individuals had more than fleeting thoughts about it. However, they are now completely happy with their initial choice.

Ultimately, our FFS patients have understood that this surgery is not to be taken lightly. They have proceeded only when they were ready. We don't proceed unless we also agree that they are ready.

Preoperative Exam and Necessary Tests

Beyond asking about your motivations and desires during that first appointment, we also take a personal and family medical history. We perform a complete physical examination, make essential facial measurements, especially with regards to proportion and symmetry. We also take and review cephalograms—specialized X-rays of the skull and jaw—CT scans, and intraoral 3-D scans of the teeth, whenever necessary. We may also order *panorex studies,* or panoramic X-rays of the teeth, sinuses, and jaw. A panorex study yields a full view of the upper and lower jaws and the temporomandibular joints.

Cephalograms remain some of the most useful imaging for recommending and planning surgery. Unlike ordinary X-rays, images from cephalograms allow the surgeon to make very precise measurements of your facial bone structure. The surgeon uses the anatomical points, planes, and angles found in a cephalogram to plot and evaluate facial size. These numbers are then evaluated against published standards.

Cone beam CT scans allow us to occasionally perform "virtual" surgical planning in cases where there is extreme asymmetry. The patient may also have anatomical features that require more precise planning than what can be accomplished with the naked eye. This type of planning adds expense to the case, and so it is used only when necessary to provide the best result.

X-Rays and Cephalograms Are Essential

To our utter amazement, we periodically hear from patients who have consulted with other surgeons or who are seeing us for "redo" surgeries and have not first had appropriate medical imaging (usually X-rays and/or cephalograms).

In our opinion, it is unsafe to perform the typical FFS forehead or jaw surgeries without the benefit of modern imaging tools. It puts the patient at substantial and unnecessary risk of serious harm. If a surgeon does not know the size and depth of the sinus and surrounding skull, the surgeon could inadvertently damage the brain. Avoid a surgeon who does not review necessary medical imaging.

We also discuss any tests we think you should undergo during your evaluation for these procedures. Anytime you have surgery, your doctor needs to have a complete understanding of your overall health. Simple screens such as a *complete blood count (CBC)* and, if necessary, an *electrocardiogram (ECG or EKG)* of your heart usually provide enough information to tell your doctor if you are healthy enough to withstand the procedure. If you have had a previous heart problem, however, a cardiac stress test may be necessary.

Other pre-op tests you may be asked to undergo include a routine chest X-ray and a blood coagulation study to gauge how your blood clots during and after surgery. You may also be asked to have a *comprehensive metabolic panel*, which can help rule out underlying medical disorders such as diabetes. Whatever tests your surgeon orders, they will be tailored to you.

Costs of the Surgery

As part of your discussion, you will no doubt want to address the financing of these surgeries. Many factors figure into the cost of facial feminization, making it difficult to offer a one-size-fits-all price without knowing the extent of the surgery. In general, however, you can plan on separate surgeon and anesthesiologist fees, along with hospital or outpatient center charges for the operating room time and staffing.

Not surprisingly, most surgeons charge more for longer operations, basing their final fees on either the total costs for all the procedures or the total time for the surgery. As you will soon learn, for instance, there are four different surgical maneuvers that we do on the forehead alone. Each one takes a different amount of time and surgical materials. After we have completely evaluated a patient, and determined a recommendation, we can then provide you with a statement describing the cost for the package of procedures you want to have performed.

Until your evaluation is complete, it is difficult to guess about the real costs of your surgery, except to say that it probably will involve a substantial out-of-pocket expense. The length of the surgery will also affect costs for an anesthesiologist and a hospital or outpatient center. These services are usually costly, and additional fees apply, based on each additional fifteen-minute segment. So, expect a higher bill for hospital facility fees when undergoing a more involved surgery. Also, you will be charged for extras, such as special materials (fixation plates and screws) and outpatient drugs (antibiotics and pain medications).

We charge a fee for an initial meeting and consultation, although many surgeons do not. A proper consultation takes a lot of time. None of our patients have complained about our modest consultation fee, because we provide a thorough evaluation and discussion.

Finally, you will have other personal costs such as travel and lodging. Most likely, none of this will be covered by health insurance.

How Many Consultations?

We certainly feel that it is not unreasonable for a patient to consult with more than one physician. It is always prudent to make sure that you feel comfortable with the professional who will be performing a potentially life-changing surgery. Yet, we question the value of visiting more than two carefully selected professionals. We find that those patients who have visited four, five, or even six different surgeons, have an inherent distrust in the professionals they consult. This is magnified by the various medical opinions they have received.

Trust is a cornerstone of a doctor–patient relationship. If a patient consults many doctors, it may indicate that he or she is a poor surgical candidate from a psychological perspective because it indicates that either the patient does not know what they want, does not know how to evaluate a surgeon, or is distrustful of the information they receive during their consultations. In any of these scenarios, the patient is not prepared for proceeding with surgery. We may, in some cases, decline to operate on those patients. Pick two trusted surgeons, and use your instinct regarding the information you receive and who to choose for your surgery.

Your Pre-op Visit

After you are scheduled for surgery, you will likely have a pre-op appointment to discuss the final plan and any concerns. Your doctor will cover a variety of steps you should take to ensure a successful operation. Although the surgeon's instructions will be tailored to your needs, below are some points to consider, especially if this is your first surgery.

Medications You'll Need to Avoid

Facial feminization involves extensive changes to your skeletal structure, so your surgeon will advise against taking drugs or preparations that may interfere with blood clotting or promote bleeding. You may need to refrain from taking these medicines before and possibly after your surgery for a certain amount of time. These include aspirin, ibuprofen, and some cardiac medications. Similarly, you will need to refrain from using supplements and herbal medications, such as omega-3, vitamin E (other than the small amount in a multivitamin), and St. John's Wort, that can potentially cause bleeding. We provide a list of specific agents that you should not be taking prior to surgery.

You may hear the same instructions regarding alcohol, which should be avoided for two weeks before surgery and two weeks after, because it can cause the blood to thin. On the other hand, you will likely receive a prescription for non-narcotic pain medication in addition to an antibiotic to help prevent infections after your surgery. We have developed a unique protocol for pain management. The result has been that very few of our patients require narcotic pain medications after surgery to maintain excellent pain control.

Other Steps You Will Want to Take

Much of the pre-op preparation for any surgery is focused on practicing good health habits. If necessary, you might be told to lose weight, control your diabetes, or get a complete physical. Your surgeon will recommend that you quit smoking prior to, and even after surgery, because smoking can increase the risk for complications. Most doctors require you quit smoking at least two weeks before your surgery. Some will not perform surgery on you unless you quit smoking.

What to Expect the Day of Surgery

Most of our patients who undergo facial feminization stay overnight in a hospital; however, smaller or single procedures can be done very safely and effectively in an outpatient environment. Operations involving an overnight stay often involve multiple procedures and complicated surgical maneuvers, so patients must initially have attentive nursing care in the unlikely event of a complication. This is especially true during the first night after surgery. Such care also makes it easier for us to check on our patients and get them started in their recovery.

We have instituted a routine practice of providing a dedicated private duty nurse to spend the night with each of our patients. It turns out that this new practice has multiple benefits for patients. This dedicated nursing care usually ensures that you will be ready to leave the hospital the day after surgery.

After you arrive at the hospital on the day of your surgery and complete the necessary paperwork, your surgeon will meet with you to discuss any final issues and answer any questions. You will also talk to the person who will provide anesthesia during your procedure. This person is usually an anesthesiologist. In other places that person might be a *certified registered nurse anesthetist (CRNA)*.

Anesthesiologists are trained to deliver various anesthetic agents, sedatives, and muscle relaxants; they also monitor your vital signs during surgery. Like your surgeon, an anesthesiologist has graduated from medical school and has completed a residency. The anesthesiologist will also have undergone fellowship training, and certainly should be board certified.

If a CRNA is providing anesthesia, that person is required to work under the supervision of an anesthesiologist. Ask who your anesthesiologist will be during your surgery and about the anesthesiologist's credentials.

The anesthesiologist will review your health history, and verify that you followed your surgeon's instructions and are ready to proceed. After you are in the operating room, your anesthesia provider will not only administer drugs in precision-measured doses, but will track your vital signs such as your heartbeat, blood pressure, and your blood oxygen saturation level.

Anesthesia

Because facial feminization involves extensive remodeling of your underlying bone structure, we prefer to perform most of our procedures under general anesthesia. As you read through this book, you will see a few exceptions to the rule. For the most part, however, we like general anesthesia because it allows us to work unencumbered for many hours while intravenous (IV) drugs and inhaled gases keep you pain free. You will be totally comfortable and safely oblivious to what is going on in the operating room.

You may be a little nervous about being unconscious, especially if we combine many procedures in one long surgery. Please rest assured that with today's anesthesia, we have been able to dramatically reduce the risks for patients. Short-acting drugs, better delivery systems, and advances in monitoring equipment, along with improved understanding of how anesthesia affects the body, allow surgeons to work safely during long procedures.

Your surgeon and anesthesia provider will ask you not to eat or drink after midnight prior to surgery. The reason is simple. On a full stomach, you risk *aspirating* or inhaling food particles into your trachea—the airway to your lungs—when you are being put under anesthesia. Because this can lead to very serious complications, your surgery will likely be postponed if you have not fasted.

Your initial anesthesia and other medications will be administered through an IV catheter inserted into a vein in your arm or hand. The catheter makes it easier to administer any intravenous antibiotics you might need during your operation. Should you require any additional medications during surgery, the catheter helps get these medicines into your system quickly and safely.

After you are prepped for surgery, you don't need to do another thing—except relax. The length of your operation depends on how many procedures you're having, and how they are grouped. If your surgery includes most of the typical FFS procedures, your surgeon will need from five to seven hours to perform the surgery. If you choose to divide your operation into two parts, you can expect to be "out" for two to four hours or more depending on the scope of the separate operations.

In the following chapters, we explain what your surgeon will be doing while you sleep comfortably. As mentioned earlier, recovery from your facial feminization procedure or procedures can take days, if not weeks. You will learn more about the effects of each procedure as you progress through this book. Keep this thought in mind: On the other side of every swollen jaw and bruised cheek will be a pleasing feminine feature.

Potential Complications with FFS Surgery

Patients often ask about the risks associated with FFS, and rightfully so. Even though this surgery is elective, it is still surgery, and usually produces permanent results. We discuss the common side effects associated with each procedure in more detail throughout this book, but there are some general risks that you should know about up front. The list that follows is by no means complete, but you need to consider these factors.

Blood Loss

A major hemorrhage during surgery is always possible, but none of our patients have experienced this complication. None of our patients have bled to the extent that a transfusion was necessary. We have had one patient who elected to have a blood transfusion the day after surgery because she lost enough blood during surgery to be somewhat anemic. Although Dr. Ousterhout has stopped two surgeries in the past because of bleeding issues, the procedures were completed a short time later and both patients did fine.

Avoiding anticoagulants, such as those for *peripheral vascular disease (PVD)*, is crucial before surgery to avoid the risk of too much blood loss. PVD can refer to disorders that affect any blood vessels. If you are on anticoagulants for a blood clotting problem, make sure you tell your doctor. Although we have never had to transfuse any of our patients during surgery, we are confident that blood from modern blood banks is screened and considered to be extremely safe for transfusions. You are more likely to be killed in a car accident driving to the hospital than to acquire a blood-borne pathogen from a blood transfusion.

Blood Clots

Traveling too soon after surgery can result in what is called a *pulmonary embolism*—a blood clot in the lungs. We give our patients exercises that will lessen this risk.

Allergic Reactions

Patients occasionally experience rashes, itching, and redness after surgery from the ointments and drugs used. These problems are rarely severe, but your surgeon will need to know if you are having problems in order to prescribe the correct treatment. After you are home, if you have any difficulty breathing, call 911 or get to a hospital immediately.

Visual Changes

Occasionally, patients complain of visual problems, such as double vision, following surgery. These issues seem to be caused by swelling or edema around the eye in the orbital area. Visual changes usually correct themselves without further treatment. None of our patients have experienced any persistent vision problems from any of these procedures.

Neuromas

Nerves are unavoidably cut during surgery, often causing temporary numbness. In the body's attempt to heal, the cut end of the nerve can develop an overgrowth called a *neuroma*.

Although neuromas are very small, they can result in an electric shock type of sensation when bumped. They usually can be treated successfully, but they also can reoccur.

Shooting Pain

It is not unusual to have brief shooting pains in your face for months, or even longer, after surgery. There is no treatment, but it is nothing to worry about. The pains will generally stop over time.

Heart Problems

Cardiac issues are always a concern during surgery. Fortunately, as noted earlier, your surgeon and anesthesiologist use high-tech monitoring equipment to keep close tabs on the way your body is responding during surgery. During Dr. Ousterhout's career, he stopped two FFS surgeries because the anesthesiologist noted an abnormality. In both cases, he was able to complete the procedures at a later date, after the patients received further treatment for their heart conditions.

Major Complications

None of our patients has ever suffered a stroke, heart attack, or death as a result of FFS. Dr. Deschamps-Braly has had one patient who had a seizure one day after surgery due to an undiagnosed medical condition. However, because the patient was admitted to the hospital, we were able to manage the situation and the patient did not have any lasting effects from the seizure. Neither of us has ever had a problem with blood clots, pressure sores, blindness, or deafness. Complications such as these are conceivable, but extremely rare.

Weakness and Fatigue

Mental and physical fatigue can be an issue for several weeks following surgery, and, on rare occasions, even months after the procedure. The weariness will disappear, sometimes suddenly. Good rest, diet, and exercise can help you get energized again.

Psychological Issues

Patients frequently suffer some level of depression after FFS procedures. Although there are too many causes to enumerate here, most episodes resolve themselves in a day or two, possibly a week. Some of our patients are already on antidepressants. If they aren't on antidepressant medications, and the depression they experience after surgery lasts longer than a week or two, it may require further treatment. Like depression, anxiety can also occur after surgery. It is often linked to the way you look after surgery, which can be disconcerting at first. You need to remind yourself to be patient. You will eventually heal.

To optimize your success with facial feminization surgery, you need to choose your surgeon wisely and prepare well, based on advice given to you by your surgeon. The more you learn about each feminization procedure, the better equipped you will be to make informed decisions. Your research will serve you very well. It will be evident in your face.

Hematomas

Hematomas are unexpected accumulations of blood underneath the skin that may require drainage if they are severe. Small hematomas may often resolve on their own or alternatively may be dealt with in the surgeon's office. However, significant hematomas may require returning to the operating room for drainage. We have had this occur only two times.

Finally, you may have sleep difficulties after surgery—until your body is free of the medications used during surgery or you have recovered from any short-term depression or are being properly treated for it.

A Final Note

Facial feminization surgery is usually a successful experience, but the road to final healing and a happy result can be difficult for some people. You will want to discuss these risks and concerns with your surgeon, who can help you through the difficult times.

3

Scalp Advancement

THE UPPER PORTION OF YOUR FACE tells the world a lot about your gender. Compared to women, men have higher hairlines, lower brows, and more thinning of their temple hair. If you want to be fully feminized, you'll need to bring your male hairline into normal female range. By lifting your brows and advancing and lowering your hairline to a more pleasing location, your surgeon can make your upper face look more feminine. This chapter explains just how *scalp advancement* can change the appearance of your upper face.

Differences in Male and Female Scalps

Physical anthropologists and other researchers have documented the significant differences in the foreheads and scalps of men and women. Through their studies, we know that the distance from the hairline down to the eyebrow at the mid-pupil line in males at age nineteen before any hair loss generally averages 6.6 cm, in contrast to about 5.08 cm in women. In most of our transgender patients, we find the distance to be closer to 7.9 cm, sometimes even more.

Although male brows in the late teens or early adulthood haven't yet dropped below the orbital or eye socket rims (as they will later in life), they still tend to be 6.35 mm or so lower than in females. In males, the eyebrows ride slightly below the bony ridge. As they age, a high percentage of young men lose hair at their temples, followed over time by loss of hair at the center of the hairline. This condition is known as a *receding hairline*. Women, on the other hand, generally do not experience thinning hair until their menopausal years. Throughout most of their lives, women's eyebrows rest above the supraorbital or upper rim of the eye socket and bony ridge of the forehead, which creates a shorter distance between their hairlines and their brows.

High hairlines and vertically long foreheads are generally accepted in males, but normally are not fashionable in females. Thus, you'll want to consider making changes to these features as part of facial feminization. Very few cisgender women with elongated foreheads pull their hair back into a ponytail, exposing a wider than average forehead length. Instead, they are

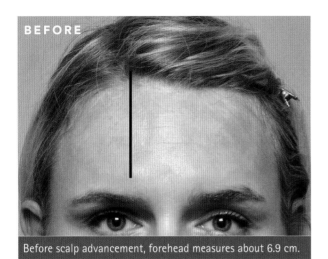

Before scalp advancement, forehead measures about 6.9 cm.

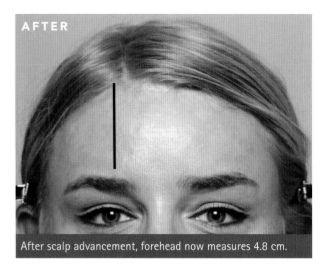

After scalp advancement, forehead now measures 4.8 cm.

likely to wear bangs, use small hairpieces, or comb their hair in other ways to camouflage the distance between their hairline and eyebrows. These women have found that sweeping their hair forward looks better than sweeping it back, which exposes a wide swath of forehead skin.

With scalp advancement and a brow lift, your surgeon can help others gender you correctly. By combining these procedures with forehead feminization, your surgeon can shorten your forehead and even minimize a receding hairline. You may no longer have to comb your hair into bangs.

Undergoing Scalp Advancement Surgery

Because scalp advancement and forehead feminization involve the same initial ear-to-ear incision, called the *coronal incision,* your plastic surgeon may recommend that these two procedures be performed at the same time. Whichever way your surgeon proceeds, advancing the scalp is usually completed under general anesthesia. If the scalp advancement is done alone, it can be completed on an outpatient basis, usually taking two or more hours

from anesthesia to recovery. If scalp advancement is combined with other facial feminization procedures, it will add an additional twenty to forty-five minutes to the operation.

Advancing the Scalp

To initiate a scalp advancement and/or forehead feminization, we usually start with an incision above the right ear. We continue the incision into the hair before moving upward toward the temple area. From there, we follow the front of the hairline, with what's known as the *pretrichial incision.* This incision can be extremely irregular or very straight, depending on the individual's current hairline shape and pattern.

After we reach the mid-forehead, we repeat the incision down to the left ear in the same fashion. Whatever the path, we place a cut just inside the hairline, angling the scalpel forward roughly forty-five degrees to preserve some follicles. This can allow the residual hair to grow through the scar and hide it. We also may remove the widow's peak if present or the patient desires it. A *widow's peak* is the descending V-shaped point at mid-hairline, which some patients prefer not to

HAIRLINE LOWERING SURGERY

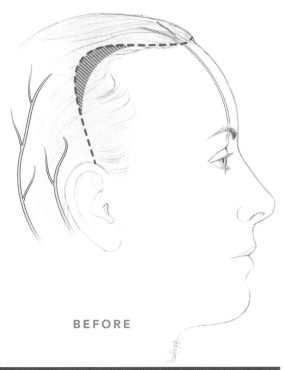

BEFORE

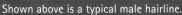

Shown above is a typical male hairline.

AFTER

A typical female hairline is about 5 cm above the eyebrows. This illustration shows how the hairline will be lowered.

have. A widow's peak looks better in males than it does in females, due to their shorter foreheads.

After the initial incision, we dissect under the scalp toward the back or far into the *occiput* or crown of the head, depending on the amount of advancement necessary. The area is then lifted, brought forward, and secured in its new position. By carefully cutting the *galea*, the thin but tight fibrous membrane covering the scalp that allows it to move as a unit, we can achieve even greater scalp advancement in patients who have higher hairlines. After we've moved and stabilized the scalp, we turn our attention to the forehead skin, elevating the eyebrows into the female position. After they are in place, we trim the excess skin before stitching the incision. The results from such surgeries have been great.

Two Scalp Surgeries May Be Necessary

Sometimes, we must tell patients that one operation to move their scalp forward or eliminate their temporal baldness will not be enough. Why? A follow-up surgery is necessary when you have extensive baldness or when there is residual hair loss in the temporal area after the first procedure. A more detailed description of a second surgery follows in the next section.

Follow-up Surgery for Extensive Hair Loss

Obviously, when men have excessive hair loss, especially at the frontal hairline, moving the scalp forward to a desired position becomes a bigger challenge. If the distance from the anterior hairline to brow, for instance, is more than 8.9 cm, a larger advancement is necessary. That is, your surgeon probably will not be able to reduce

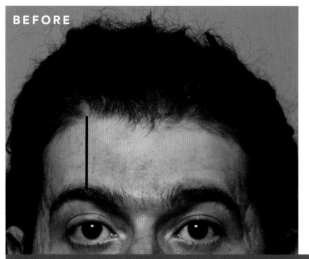

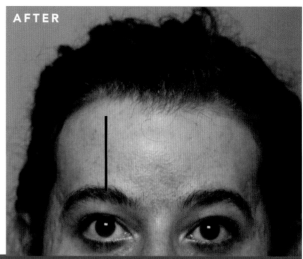

BEFORE

AFTER

This patient underwent a scalp elevation (the opposite of what is typically performed) in order to move her hairline height to a more feminine position.

this much baldness in a single operation. Two or more scalp advancements will be necessary.

We usually don't carry out the second advancement until a year has passed after the first surgery. By then, the residual scalp has become looser and is ready for further advancement. Right after the first operation, the scalp is tight. As will be discussed later, we prescribe Rogaine for our patients after both of these surgeries to help prevent hair loss secondary to the tension on the scalp. These procedures must be completed under general anesthesia.

There are other additional, yet less practical, procedures that may be performed in cases of severe hair loss. For instance, expansion of areas of the scalp may be accomplished using slowly inflating balloons beneath the skin. This is a very slow method to allow for stretching and removal of skin that contains no hair. Yet, this laborious procedure is often impractical for many people and most choose to wear a hairpiece instead. However, it is an option for those who want it.

Residual Temporal Baldness after Scalp Advancement

If you have rather severe hair loss at your temples, your surgeon can use scalp advancement to bring the mid-anterior or front hairline into a female position. The areas of baldness at your temples will not be totally eliminated with this initial procedure, although they will be reduced. Why? The scalp can only be stretched in one direction at a time, similar to a rubber band pulled tightly.

We frequently complete additional procedures to reduce large areas of temporal baldness even more. We can usually eliminate an additional 12.7 mm of scalp skin with each secondary advancement. In a few patients with extremely large areas of temporal baldness, we have even performed as many as four additional advancements. But there is an important caveat to consider: Follow-up surgeries are limited reductions that can only be completed four or more months after the previous surgery.

It is financially beneficial for you to undergo scalp advancement as opposed to transplanting hairs. Keep in mind, however, that there is a point of diminishing returns with secondary scalp advancement for temporal baldness. At some time, usually not until the second or third additional surgery, some people find it fiscally wiser to consider hair transplants for any remaining area of baldness. Hair transplants can be costly and time-consuming because each follicle is transplanted one at a time. You need to weigh this cost and time commitment against the expense and time needed for secondary advancements.

Hairline Position Based on Height

The position of the final front hairline is based to a degree of an individual's height. In a five-foot-six to five-foot-seven female, for instance, the hairline generally rides about 5 cm above the top of the eyebrows. In scalp advancement, we generally reduce that distance slightly during surgery because the skin will likely stretch a few millimeters in the first two months after surgery.

Because we know that the brow will drop after surgery, we overcorrect it slightly during the procedure. Obviously, the height is increased in taller individuals and decreased in shorter people. Occasionally, patients are happy with a longer forehead because they've seen it in other women. But in most transfeminine individuals, the finished forehead length is proportional to their height and other features.

Correcting Previous Surgeries

Can a surgeon correct a long forehead resulting from previous forehead or brow lift surgery? Yes. Many patients need scalp advancement because a prior operation left them with an elongated forehead. Correcting such a long forehead, however, is not always easy. The original incision

across the top of the head is often within the hair, usually far forward and close to the hairline. As a result, the surgeon performing the secondary procedure doesn't have much leeway to make the necessary pre-hairline incision without skin or hair loss.

When patients ask for an additional scalp advancement, we have to position the second cut directly in front of the hairline. This leaves limited circulation to the hair and scalp between the two cuts. Because blood does not travel well across a scar, there is a risk of losing some scalp as a result of tissue death.

The loss of scalp depends on the potential space between the incisions and the time between the initial surgery and follow-up surgeries. If the distance between the incisions is less than a centimeter, we use the old scar and excise or cut out the narrow strip of hair in front of it before advancing the scalp. If the area of scalp between the two incisions is larger than 2 cm, we create a new pre-hairline incision, hoping to preserve the hair-bearing scalp between the two incisions.

Again, our choices and chances for success depend on the time between the procedures. If the first operation was completed at least eighteen months to two years beforehand, we are less worried about losing part of the scalp from lack of blood supply. If the first operation was not within this time frame, we have a real concern. In either case, the goal is to reposition the scalp into a female position and preserve your hair.

The other problem we encounter with previous procedures, is that some surgeons put the lower ends of their pre-hairline incisions in the temporal or temple hair. Because the hair in that area is thin, the scar will almost always show. Hair transplants to cover any cuts in this area

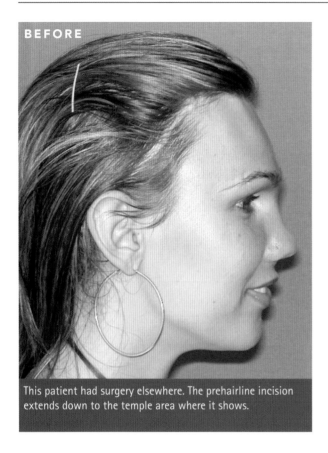

This patient had surgery elsewhere. The prehairline incision extends down to the temple area where it shows.

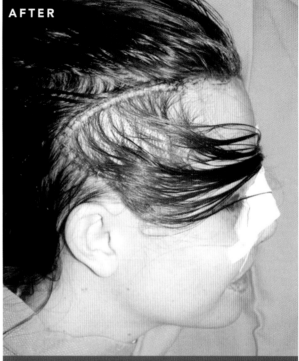

This postoperative photo shows my preferred temporal and prehairline incision for scalp advancement and forehead contouring. This incision will be hidden.

are much more difficult to achieve because of the angle at which the hair grows out of the scalp.

Even worse, if the first surgeon has made the incision in front of the temple hair, an unsightly scar along the edge of the hairline can occur. There's no need for this kind of outcome because a scalp advancement incision can be placed farther back to the ear, well hidden by thicker hair. When such scars occur, a combination of permanent cosmetic tattoos and hair transplants are often helpful to improve the appearance.

After Your Scalp Advancement Surgery

Patients undergoing scalp advancement have every reason to expect a good recovery. Because this surgery is generally completed on an inpatient basis with other surgeries, most individuals spend one night in the hospital following the procedure. Most of your recovery, however, will take place at home. To maximize results and keep you complication free, you'll need to know the following information about recovery from scalp advancement surgery.

Recovery Follow-up Care

After surgery, you'll leave the operating room with stitches in the pre-hairline area and staples in your scalp. Your surgeon will have removed both the stitches and staples by the fourth to sixth day post-op. If you're having other procedures simultaneously, such as nose or chin feminizations, you'll have supporting dressings so you'll need to be extra cautious when you shower. We recommend waiting to shampoo your hair until your first postoperative appointment.

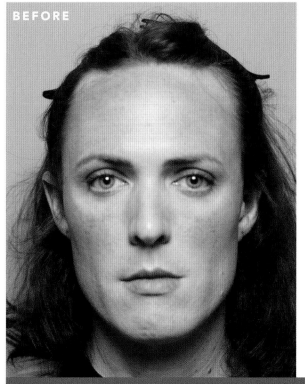

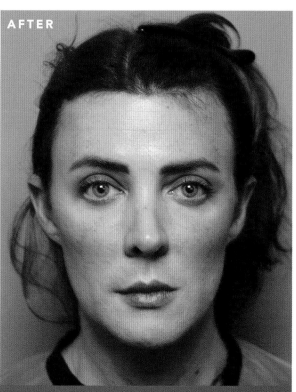

This patient underwent forehead contouring (Type III), scalp advancement (hairline lowering), brow lift, rhinoplasty, genioplasty (chin reshaping), jaw tapering (jaw reduction/feminization), gonial angle resection (removal of the back corners of the jaw), and fat grafting (volume addition to the cheeks, under eyes, lips, and perioral area).

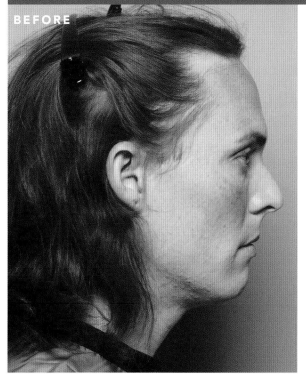

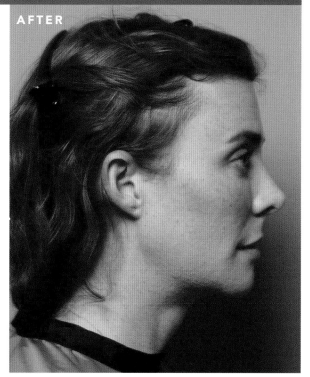

Refrain from using any hair dyes or treatments for at least six weeks after the scabs along your scalp incision fall off. Because numbness may be an issue, you should not use the heat settings on your hair dryer for at least a month after surgery. After surgery, because you won't have sensation immediately, you will not feel how hot things such as a blow-dryer are on the skin. Your normal protection mechanisms that tell you to stop doing something because it is too hot will not be working. Therefore, you can burn your scalp quite easily. This is why you should be careful after scalp advancement surgery when styling your hair. Swelling and bruising around the eyes should be gone within ten to twelve days after the surgery.

Most patients can return to their usual activities within seven days, especially if they work from home. But don't overly exert yourself for three weeks after the surgery. Don't do anything that causes you to sweat or raise your blood pressure.

However, we recommend significant amounts of walking very early after surgery. In our experience, walking tends to help relieve some of the swelling that results from surgery. It can also help clear from the system the remaining anesthetic agents that cause one to feel sluggish after a surgical procedure.

Pain Medications, Antibiotics, and Other Treatments

With scalp advancement, there is minimal discomfort, so you probably will need nothing more than non-narcotic pain relievers for a few days. Infections are extremely rare, but you will be placed on antibiotics, especially if you're having additional procedures.

Many products on the market today claim to enable healing so that you won't see your scar. Do not use them. These formulations can cause hair loss along the sides of the incision. *A word to the wise:* Don't put anything on your scalp unless your surgeon approves it.

Side Effects and Potential Complications of Scalp Advancement

Scalp advancement is a well-tolerated surgery. Still, be aware that you will have a scar, temporary numbness, and even elevated brows after the operation. You may also have hair issues, which we will discuss later. But first, here are a few of the more common concerns related to scalp advancement.

Scars

If placed correctly, scalp advancement scars are very acceptable and not even noticeable in most patients. Many surgeons have said they do not do this procedure because it leaves a very

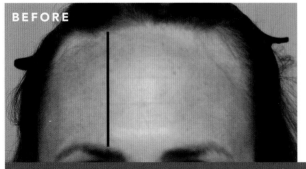
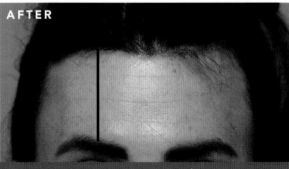

Before and after surgery. The hairline was reduced by 2 cm (as measured between the eyebrows and the hairline).

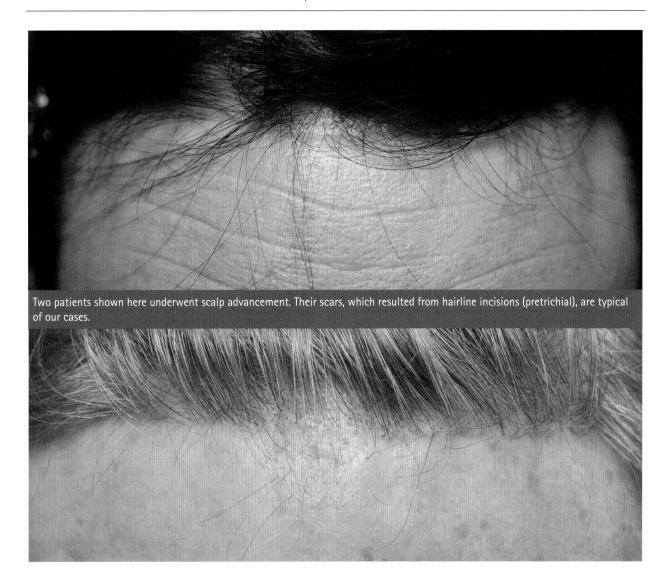

Two patients shown here underwent scalp advancement. Their scars, which resulted from hairline incisions (pretrichial), are typical of our cases.

noticeable scar. The doctors who say this, may lack the skills and experience needed for scalp advancement surgery.

Scars are simply nature's way of healing, so they are not bad in and of themselves. If the residual scar bothers any of our patients after scalp advancement, we may do further surgery if we feel that it can produce improvements. Otherwise, we recommend placing a few hair transplants directly into the area of any visible scar. Normally, the result is very nice.

Elevated Brows

One of the issues in combining scalp advancement with forehead feminization and brow lift, is that a patient will end up with a temporary startled look because of the initial position where the brows are placed. The brows drop down into a more normal position between one and two months post-surgery.

Numbness

Temporary numbness occurs with scalp advancement surgery because two sensory nerves, the supraorbital nerves, are unavoidably cut during the procedure. Patients will almost always experience a short-term loss of sensation in a fist-size area atop the head. Although 1 to 2 percent of these individuals may never regain their full sensation (similar to accidents and major surgery), the remaining 98 percent will recover normal to near-normal feeling in twelve to eighteen months. Why? Because the supraorbital nerves which flank the forehead and stimulate the scalp regenerate, or more sensory nerves in the area take over. So, chances are good that you will feel the top of your head again. In time, you probably will forget that it was even a problem.

Your surgeon may try to convince you that an endoscopic approach—moving the tissue through a keyhole incision with fiber-optic instruments—will produce the same result without skin loss or numbness. In our experience, this approach does not work for scalp advancement. One cannot achieve scalp advancement without a coronal incision. To bring the scalp forward, you must excise or remove some of the forehead skin. It will not shrink with an endoscopic approach as some surgeons claim.

Long-term numbness is rare with scalp advancement, so this side effect is not a reason to avoid the procedure. The results are too good.

Motor Nerve Paralysis

Paralysis of the *seventh cranial* or *facial nerve* is an extremely rare event after scalp advancement. The seventh cranial nerve comes out of the skull behind and beneath the ear and proceeds underneath the *parotid gland,* the major salivary gland that swells when you get the mumps. There, it branches into the neck, face, and forehead to perform motor functions. Two branches wind their way to the forehead, where they lift your brows in surprise or lower and bring them together for a frown or questioning look. We have never experienced a seventh nerve injury from dissecting the scalp or lifting the forehead during a primary surgery. This outcome is possible, however, so we discuss it with every patient. If nerve damage occurs, it's not a given that the nerve will regenerate, but chances are, it will come back.

Temporary Hair Loss

Advancing your scalp can help you address or even eliminate your receding hairline because the scalp is moved forward. But there can also be temporary hair loss at the incision or in the scalp tissue itself with this procedure. We have found that if hair loss is going to occur, it usually surfaces during the first month and a half after surgery. After the initial period of hair loss, there is usually no hair growth for another six months. Just around the time the patient gives up hope that hair will return, whiskers begin to surface. After that, the hair usually returns fully.

Any potential hair loss will depend on a variety of factors, but the amount of baldness you're trying to correct, is probably the most important. In general, the more widespread the baldness, the more tension there is, on the scalp from the advancement. Greater tension on the scalp also heightens the risk for increased hair loss after surgery. Other factors affecting hair loss include the natural growth and state of your hair, the hormones you may be taking for your transition, and whether or not you are using hair restoration drugs such as Rogaine.

When we know that one of our patients will need larger scalp advancement, we start that person on Rogaine at least one day before surgery. The patient also needs to continue taking Rogaine for at least three months afterward.

This regimen seems to help prevent further hair loss in patients who already have extreme baldness. Sometimes, however, hair is lost on each side of the incision, which I attribute to tension on the skin. Rarely is this type of loss permanent. If it is, the loss can usually be improved through a scar revision. If residual loss still occurs, however, we suggest hair transplants.

Complete Hair Loss Is Rare but Possible

Complete hair loss after scalp advancement or forehead surgery is extremely rare, but it does occur. During our many years in practice, only one transfeminine patient lost all her hair after scalp advancement. She thought it was due to the surgery, but the loss included areas of her body that were not involved in the operation. The back of her scalp, for instance, was bare, which had nothing to do with the front of her scalp, the area of the procedure. We assured her that her hair would come back, which it did in time.

Rarely, some people are so stressed by surgery, that they sustain a temporary loss of hair. Is this a routine reaction? Not at all. Fortunately, it seems to occur only in people who are extremely worried about their operation.

Hair Restoration Medications

Although moving your scalp forward can create a fuller hairline, it may not partially or fully resolve baldness. Then, your options begin with, but are not limited to, hair restoration drugs.

Hair restoration drugs such as Rogaine *(minoxidil)*, Propecia *(finasteride)*, and Avodart *(dutasteride)* are helping many people deal with pattern hair loss *(alopecia)*. These medications are also very effective for stimulating hair growth before and after scalp advancement surgery.

If you have not undergone gender confirmation surgery or an *orchiectomy* (removal of your testicles), you may benefit from a topical solution or other medications, especially if receding hairlines and baldness run in your family. These medicines may preserve your existing hair and prevent further loss. If you have already undergone GCS, you won't have the same hair worries as you did in your assigned gender, because your body will no longer be producing as much testosterone. Keep in mind, however, that even with the best results, you will need a scalp advancement to obtain a feminine hairline if you are transitioning.

One caveat, however: Our experience with many patients suggests that there is an age limit when it comes to the effectiveness of some of today's hair restoration medications. After you reach age fifty, you probably won't be successful in stimulating new hair growth with medications such as Propecia or Avodar, at either the top of your head or frontal hairline area.

Rogaine

An over-the-counter topical solution applied to the scalp twice a day, Rogaine *(minoxidil)* reinvigorates shrunken hair follicles, increases their size, and helps regrow thicker hair over time. Its active ingredient is minoxidil, a vasodilator known for relaxing coronary arteries and veins.

Rogaine works best for restoring hair at the crown or top back of the head. It doesn't work as well for stimulating the temple area, although it does help prevent further hair loss. We recommend Rogaine, which the pharmaceutical company Upjohn introduced in 1988, when patients are undergoing larger scalp advancements. The reason is that Rogaine helps prevent hair loss connected to the increased skin tension with scalp advancement.

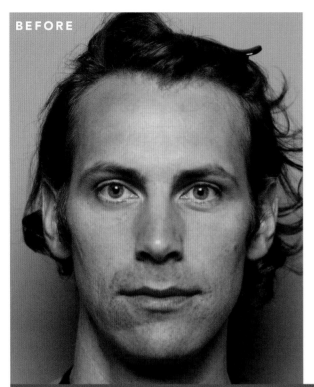

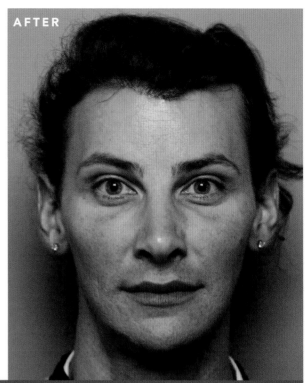

This patient underwent forehead contouring (Type III), orbital reshaping, scalp advancement (hairline lowering), brow lift, feminizing rhinoplasty, fat grafting (fat injections throughout the face), upper lip lift (shortening), chin osteotomy (chin reshaping), and jaw contouring.

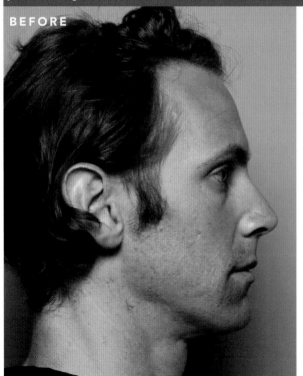

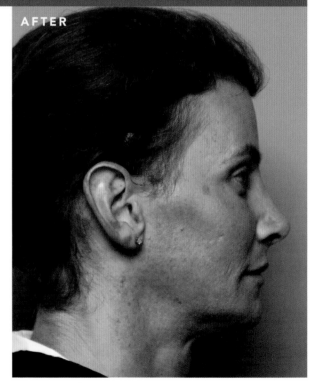

Propecia

Since it was introduced in 1997, Propecia (*finasteride*) has proven to be very effective for male pattern baldness on the top of the head. There is insufficient evidence, however, that it works for receding hairlines. Propecia is taken in a one-milligram pill once daily. It restores hair by preventing the conversion of testosterone into *DHT (dihydrotestosterone)*, a chemical involved in both hair loss and *benign prostatic hyperplasia (BPH)*, an enlarged prostate. (BPH is treated with drugs containing the same active ingredient, finasteride.)

Some studies suggest that after three years of using Propecia, it is more than 75 percent effective in blocking *5-alpha reductase*, the enzyme responsible for dihydrotestosterone (DHT) formulation, at the hair follicle site. If your hairline is actively receding, some doctors advise patients to combine Rogaine and Propecia for a year because the combination seems to work better than either treatment alone.

Avodart

Another oral drug for treating enlarged prostate, Avodart *(dutasteride),* has also shown great success for male pattern baldness. Its active ingredient, dutasteride, is more effective than any other drug in preventing the conversion of testosterone to DHT. A generic version, sold under the name *dutasteride,* is now available. Some reports suggest that it is more than 95 percent effective in inhibiting the enzymes responsible for DHT formulation at the hair follicle. We believe Avodart is the drug of choice for hair loss, even though the medication is currently only prescribed for BPH. A 0.5-milligram-per-day pill to address hair loss is an off-label use, meaning doctors can prescribe it, but it has not received official FDA approval for preventing hair loss.

Spironolactone

Spironolactone is a potassium-sparing diuretic that blocks the actions of *aldosterone,* a hormone that regulates the body's balance of water and salt. Prescribing it for alopecia is an off-label use of this medicine. It blocks production of androgens and the effect of androgen at receptor sites. Its side effects include *gynecomastia* or overdevelopment of the male breast, so its use has been limited for male pattern baldness. In the transgender population, however, it works quite well.

Cimetidine

The drug *Cimetidine* is an H-2 antagonist used to treat acid reflux and peptic ulcers. Prescribing it as an anti-androgen for patients with hair loss is an off-label use.

Hair Transplants

There are several situations in which hair transplants are useful. Most of our patients are extremely pleased with the scar resulting from scalp advancement. It heals very well, blending nicely with the surrounding skin. But in some individuals, the wound doesn't mend exactly as predicted, or the natural angle of the hair makes the scar more obvious. In these cases, we recommend hair transplants.

In other situations, replacing the lost follicles with grafts harvested from the back of the head works well to replenish a balding crown or receding hairline. Why so? When hair grafts are transplanted, they grow in the same way as they did in their original location. That is, if your hair is growing fully along your collar, it should grow nicely at your hairline or on your crown.

You will find details on hair transplants in chapter 15.

Hair Transplants during Your Facial Feminization Surgery

We have performed hair transplants during the primary facial feminization surgery approximately a dozen times. Our experience has led us to abandon this procedure for a number of reasons. The hair transplants do not live nearly as well if transplanted at the time of the primary surgery as compared when they are performed six months later as a second independent operation. Secondly, we do not feel doing hair transplants during scalp advancement surgery provides good value to the patient who is paying for general anesthesia in addition to the hair transplants.

Chapter 15 focuses on hair transplants and describes the considerations, options, and outcomes for hair transplants. Hair transplants should not be taken from areas of the head, such as the top of the scalp, that are prone to thinning. Rather, hair grafts should be taken from the back of the scalp. However, harvesting hair grafts from the back of the scalp is not an option during FFS surgery. The reason for this is it requires a second incision in the back of the scalp which can compromise the circulation to the top of the scalp.

In addition, if a coronal incision is used at the back of the head, invariably the hairline will slide upward and higher on your forehead during closure of the coronal incision. It is, to say the least, counterintuitive to slide someone's hairline upward only to use hair transplants to then lower it. This would result in an unnatural-appearing hairline that is thinner than one's natural hair should be providing.

Undergoing hair transplantation during FFS surgery may be a good idea for someone who would prefer not to waste hair that might be removed during scalp advancement and temporal lift if it fits your budget. Yet, hair transplanted this way—while the scalp is under tension—may not survive as well as hair harvested during a separate procedure. The survival rate for hair grafts transplanted during FFS is 60 percent of the survival rate for those grafts harvested in a separate procedure.

If you are planning scalp advancement surgery, hold off on any transplants beforehand. Transplants should ideally be done after your scalp advancement. Also, previously placed hair implants may end up being removed during surgery, making them a waste of money. If a bald spot on the crown is your only worry, you can take care of that anytime.

The other issue with doing hair transplants before surgical scalp advancement is that the scar across the back of the head from the hair transplants may create circulation problems later, which compromise the necessary blood supply to the front of the scalp at the time of formal scalp advancement. Therefore, hair transplants should be delayed until after your recovery from feminization surgery.

Outcome of Scalp Advancement Surgery

Scalp advancement results are generally so good, that patients actually get a tremendous psychological lift from undergoing this procedure. It gives most individuals a normal feminine hair pattern and density not possible with hair transplants or other hair replacement methods alone. (Even after three transplant sessions, for instance, the density is still only one-third to one-half normal thickness.) It's hard to say which facial feminization surgery gives individuals the most satisfaction because they all go hand in hand. But for people with long foreheads and some hairline baldness, scalp advancement is a satisfying, worthwhile procedure.

Commonly Asked Questions

I have a high forehead, but I do not want to risk any numbness at the hairline from an elective surgery. Can you feminize my face without scalp advancement? Yes, but not completely. All of the facial feminization procedures mentioned in this book are optional. But shortening the height of the forehead is one of the most important steps you can take in your facial transition from male to female. It's as important as reshaping your forehead and reducing your thyroid cartilage, two other giveaways of your assigned gender.

Don't let the rare, albeit possible, chance of permanent numbness, prevent you from undergoing this surgery. Lack of sensation is not a significant long-term issue. Also consider this: If you are undergoing a forehead feminization, your surgeon will need to get to the forehead bone through the same coronal incision across your scalp. That means the surgeon is already in a position to advance the scalp. What you do is up to you, but all objective evidence dictates that to get the best facial feminization result, you will want scalp advancement.

Will scalp advancement cause me to lose hair sooner? We have not seen this among our patients. Some individuals, however, continue to lose their hair after gender reassignment surgery. If you have any hair-loss issues, talk to your doctor. Medications such as Rogaine may help.

I do not want a pre-hairline scar, but I have a long forehead. What can I do? Your choices, unfortunately, are limited. A good surgeon will do everything to minimize the scar. If even a small scar would be unsatisfactory, however, you may have to accept having a long forehead.

The only hair on my head is along the back of my skull. I do not want to wear a hairpiece. What else can I do? If you are younger than age fifty, try a hair-stimulating medication, such as Avodart. If after twelve months you haven't seen significant regrowth, you may have no choice but to consider a hairpiece. In fact, if you are older than age fifty, you will need one for sure.

When should I start medication to help restore my hair? You should start as soon as your lack of hair becomes a visual concern. If you are having scalp advancement or forehead surgery, however, consult with your surgeon before trying anything.

All of my brothers have bald heads. Will I lose my hair, as well? Heredity is hard to predict; all brothers are not alike. The inheritance pattern is usually through maternal grandfathers. In other words, if you look more like your mother, or her father, and he had hair, you might not lose yours.

A Final Note

Bringing your hairline into female range can change the entire way your upper face appears to the world. By moving your scalp forward, your surgeon can reduce your forehead height and relocate your brows into a more desirable female position. In the process, your receding hairline will hopefully be totally eliminated.

Performed in conjunction with forehead feminization (explained in the chapter 4), scalp advancement is an essential step in achieving your feminine appearance. This procedure, along with chin reduction, also makes the vertical dimension of the face appear smaller, which is necessary to produce a feminine result.

FFS PATIENT PROFILE: Sally

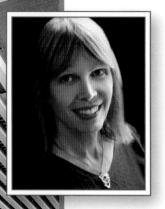

Sally is a retired defense contractor who had facial feminization when she was forty-three. Dr. Douglas Ousterhout performed her surgery.

WHEN DID YOU BEGIN THINKING ABOUT TRANSITIONING? WHAT WAS MOTIVATING YOUR DESIRE TO TRANSITION?

I was a teenager when I realized transition through surgery was possible, but for many years afterward, I thought transition was for others, not me. I was convinced that I was far too masculine to be able to make my life work as a woman. Then at age thirty-six, I finally could no longer take the frustration of living as the wrong gender. Through the internet, I contacted others with similar stories and began to learn what was possible. I did not want to live my life as a man playing at being a woman. When I saw what Dr. Ousterhout could do, I realized that physical limitations were no longer a barrier to my own transition.

WHAT PROCEDURES DID YOU HAVE PERFORMED?

I underwent forehead feminization, eyebrow lift, rhinoplasty, chin advancement and tapering, jaw reduction, and masseter muscle reduction, which reduced the fullness of my jawline.

WHICH PROCEDURES WERE PERFORMED SIMULTANEOUSLY AND WHICH ONES WERE STAGED?

I had all my procedures done on the same day in July 1999.

HOW WOULD YOU DESCRIBE YOUR SURGICAL EXPERIENCES? DID YOU HAVE MUCH PAIN? WHAT WAS THE RECOVERY LIKE?

I was miserable for a few days, but through the miracle of well-managed drugs, I felt very little pain. It was more like the discomfort of having the flu. For the first couple of days, I was very weak and tired. I could only breathe through my mouth (due to nasal packing) for several days and sleeping was a challenge. The biggest relief was when the nose packing came out. By the end of the first week, I was getting out and about without difficulty.

As I healed, the biggest problem was numbness in my lower face, which took a few weeks to disappear. My nose took some months to completely heal, and numbness in my skull actually persisted for several years before it felt normal. After the bandages came off, I was able to cover some residual bruising effectively with makeup and I looked fine.

HOW DO YOU FEEL THE FFS SURGERY AFFECTED THE WAY OTHERS PERCEIVE YOU AND THE WAY YOU PERCEIVE YOURSELF?

When the bandages were removed, the effect was immediate and profound. Without hesitation, others perceived me as a woman. I needed no makeup or feminine clothing for this to happen. Once timid in public, I now felt I had a pass to confidently go anywhere.

WHAT ADVICE WOULD YOU OFFER TO OTHERS WHO ARE CONSIDERING FFS?

Do not underestimate how important FFS can be to a successful transition. FFS enabled me to navigate confidently through a very conservative professional environment and keep my career intact. Building new social relationships was simplified, and I quickly integrated into a new life as a woman. I strongly believe things would have been quite difficult without the surgery.

FFS is very complex, difficult, and expensive surgery. For many people, significant bone work is required and traditional, more superficial cosmetic procedures will not be satisfactory. A facelift might make you look younger, but it won't make you look like a woman. Get a good assessment of your needs, understand what procedures will be required, and choose your surgeon accordingly.

Finally, realize that FFS isn't for everyone. Thousands of transgender women transition successfully without it. Some people are fortunate and their faces are not heavily masculine. Other women feel no need for facial feminization and are able to live as they wish. But for those like myself, FFS offered hope, and after a lifetime of despair, it felt like a true miracle. I will always be grateful to Dr. Doug Ousterhout, his assistant Mira Colluccio, and staff for enabling me to live the life I had given up as beyond reach.

LOOKING BACK OVER TWENTY YEARS AFTER FACIAL FEMINIZATION, WHAT DO YOU THINK ABOUT YOUR CHOICE IN RETROSPECT?

I had a bit of rose-colored glasses on going into this. I don't think I really appreciated the seriousness of the procedures and what some of the risks entailed, particularly possible permanent nerve damage. I have a chin implant, and once in awhile if I rest my chin on my fist in a specific way, I might feel it pinch a little bit.

I was numb on the top of my head for years. It took quite awhile to settle out. It was a number of years before it felt like it was really gone. I have feeling up there now, but I can still feel some kind of tightness or something if I tighten my head muscles. It's not annoying and it doesn't impede me. It's just a reminder of that feeling. Maybe there are still some numb places and I've gotten used to it and just over-mapped it. The nose took awhile to settle, too. I had a lot of nasal dryness and bloody noses.

There's nothing now that's an annoyance, and nothing that I would consider a long-term adverse side effect.

IN WHAT LONG-TERM WAYS DID FFS CHANGE YOUR LIFE?

When I transitioned, I was in an extremely conservative environment with the military intelligence community. Very quickly I could tell my employer was assessing me and my employability threshold. I think FFS gave me the ability to go into work environments where I wasn't going to draw attention to myself as an obviously transgender person. I was able to fly under the radar in that environment within a couple of months after transitioning. I think it would have been very different otherwise.

I realize how loaded that can be today with "passing privilege," but that was my experience in 1999. I was working in Brussels at NATO for a U.S. company. After I came out to my family, I went to corporate headquarters and presented the head of HR with a binder of information. The next day she told me, "I talked to legal and we could fire you, but we're going to do the right thing." The CEO reviewed my binder and credentials and said, "I could use a few hundred resumes like this." I had been advised by a friend that I needed a bellwether person to help me succeed, and the HR director ended up being that, and the CEO backed her.

I was lucky, but the combination of my good preparation and my appearance and ability to navigate the social situations were also key. We agreed on my transfer to Washington, DC, where they stuck me in a back office while they tried to figure out what to do with me. I was soon assigned as project lead on a counterintelligence project, but they would not let me do a company-wide announcement. So, I would encounter people who didn't realize I was someone they had met before.

The project required working with government people directly to determine needs and find technical solutions. That required me to be out there with them day to day. It was pretty clear that I was not perceived as trans because I would occasionally hear transphobic comments that were clearly not directed at me. That was soul withering, but I was not in a position at that time to speak out. When I turned fifty, after several promotions, my partner and I chucked it all, bought a sailboat, and literally sailed away.

FFS really was an investment, because it allowed me to sustain my career, retire early, and do stuff I wanted to do. I haven't felt a need to have anything done since then, and the surgery I had over twenty years ago, still serves me well today.

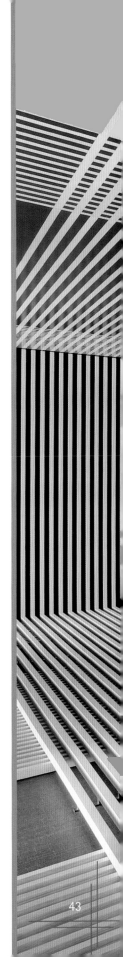

4

Forehead Feminization

YOU CAN EASILY TELL the difference between men and women by their foreheads. Perhaps no other facial feature, other than your Adam's apple, distinguishes your masculinity quite like this part of your face. Males exhibit greater hooding over their eyes, greater *bossing* (or roundness) under their eyebrows, and greater overall forward projection than females.

Because your forehead's contour is an obvious sign of your assigned gender, modifying the primary elements is an important step in your feminization. Given the right surgeon and proper surgical approach, recontouring your forehead can dramatically change your appearance. Our objective is to not only help you look better, but to help you look your very best.

Differences in the Male and Female Foreheads

The forehead covers a large portion (from 20 to 40 percent) of the face, and the forehead displays a markedly different contour and projection in men compared to women. Most people don't pay attention to how their forehead is shaped or even how it protrudes from the face. Yet, physical anthropologists have been studying these very features for centuries and have long recognized the distinctions between the sexes. In their seminal anthropology book, *From Lucy to Language,* authors Donald Johanson and Blake Edgar introduce male and female skulls dating back several million years, based on specific gender characteristics.

Male foreheads are defined by three factors: a significant forward projection; a pronounced roundness, called *brow bossing*, just above the eyes; and a flat or hollow spot about 2.5 cm above the bridge of the nose. Females have little or no bossing. Their foreheads tend to be rounded, with smooth, even surfaces.

Unlike women, men have more hooding and additional fullness at the superior lateral angle of the orbit—the area directly to the outside of the eye socket's upper skeletal rim. Male foreheads also project farther forward in front of the eyes than do female foreheads. This projection can be even more pronounced in males who exhibit larger-than-normal frontal sinuses, referred to as *hyperpneumatization*.

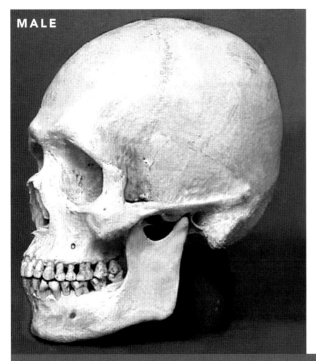
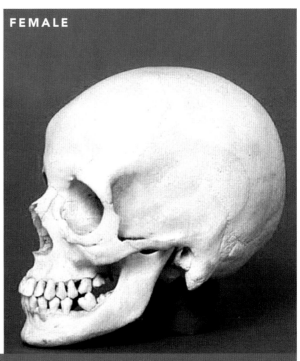

MALE

FEMALE

Feminization of the male forehead involves eliminating the fullness of the male brow ridge on the skull.

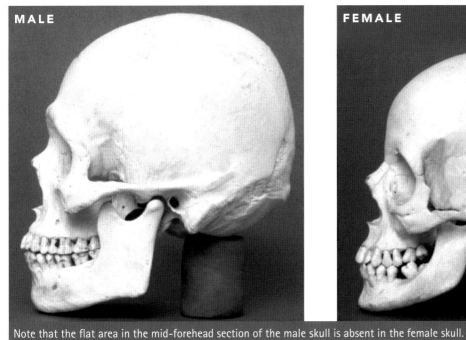
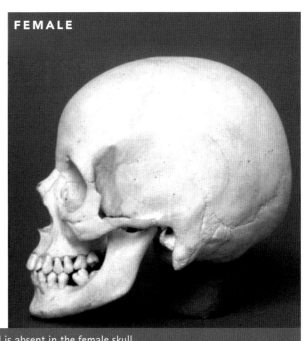

MALE

FEMALE

Note that the flat area in the mid-forehead section of the male skull is absent in the female skull.

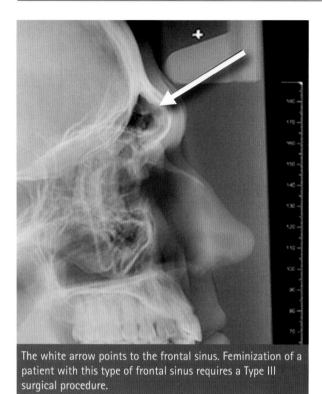

The white arrow points to the frontal sinus. Feminization of a patient with this type of frontal sinus requires a Type III surgical procedure.

The *frontal sinuses* are a pair of air-filled cavities in the mid-lower forehead above the nose and eyes, and they lessen the skeletal load of your skull. Frontal sinuses vary tremendously in size from nonexistent to very large. Is there a correlation between the extent of forehead bossing and the extent of the sinuses? Not necessarily.

Even though men with average or greater frontal bossing do have frontal sinuses, men with less prominent bossing may or may not have them. (Surprisingly, 5 percent of people lack frontal sinuses; 8 percent only have one sinus.) They may still have a male forehead contour, however. Because your frontal sinuses have nothing to do with voice or voice resonance, reducing them (as we do in one forehead feminization approach called *Type III*) won't have any impact on the pitch of your voice.

Unfortunately, your voice won't go from a bass viola to a violin.

The size of your frontal sinuses rarely makes the male forehead significantly less masculine or a female forehead less feminine than what's normal for each gender.

Ethnicity Makes a Difference

Significant ethnic differences are apparent in brow-forehead prominence. African American foreheads are generally less prominent than those of Caucasians. Chinese and Korean foreheads, however, show considerably less prominence than Caucasians. Japanese foreheads in particular are situated so far back, that the forehead is located behind the prominence of the eye in many cases. It is even more complicated to describe the brow-forehead prominence among individuals of mixed ethnicity or race. Regardless of your ethnicity, your surgeon should be able to customize a forehead feminization procedure for you.

Undergoing Forehead Feminization Surgery

Our goal in performing forehead feminization is not only to eliminate any hint of masculinity in our transfeminine patients, but also to make them as attractive as possible. It is not enough to burr down or shave the brow prominence a millimeter or two before getting into the frontal sinus. We have seen this approach fail in people who've come to us for a secondary surgery following an unsuccessful first attempt by another surgeon.

In the great majority of these individuals, the anterior (front) wall of the frontal sinus was not sufficiently thick to allow an adequate reduction before the bone was burred all the way into the frontal sinus. Our objective with these patients—and all of our patients—is to make sure that we use the best approach possible for their unique forehead needs.

Forehead Feminization Approaches

The first male-to-female (MTF) individual referred to Dr. Ousterhout was in 1982, for forehead feminization. By that time, he had been performing craniofacial surgery for many years at the University of California, San Francisco Medical School. Yet, craniofacial surgery at the time was primarily focused on correcting congenital problems, rather than correcting gender incongruence. Dr. Ousterhout had never been required to focus so closely on the measurement differences between male and female skulls. Before he attempted the surgery, he studied multiple texts on facial physical anthropology and examined approximately 2,000 skulls, many of which were part of the Atkinson Skull Collection of the University of the Pacific School of Dentistry.

Based on this research, he formulated and defined four operations which he labeled as *Type I, Type II, Type III,* and *Type IV.* These categories address various skull issues that must be overcome to obtain a more feminized forehead. These issues include the protrusion or prominence of the brows, the presence and size of the sinuses, the thickness of the frontal sinus wall, and the thickness of the anterior or frontal skull (just above the sinuses). The surgeon must also address the curvature and slant of the forehead and the depth of the concavity or depression just above the brow bossing.

Many surgeons who perform FFS are content to burr away only a small amount of bone either directly or endoscopically from the forehead and call it a feminization. With an endoscope, a surgeon makes an incision and inserts a tiny camera, which then guides the surgeon's movements. But the many potential variations in the human skull

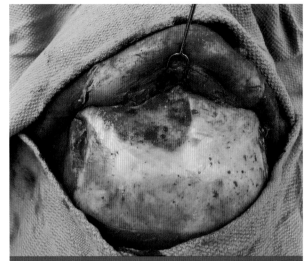

Photo shows Type I forehead feminization being performed. Bone thickness is being reduced by approximately 1 cm. Patient's orbital rims, upper edges of the eye sockets, are also being contoured.

prohibit relying solely on one operation. Burring alone is totally insufficient in 95 percent of cases.

Dr. Ousterhout's research and the four resulting approaches he first developed, have been effective for more than thirty years. In all these surgeries, the objective is to eliminate the bossing and hooding above the eyes, to place the forehead protrusion in an appropriate female position, and to create the most aesthetically pleasing forehead contour possible.

To do so, we initiate every surgery through a *coronal incision,* the incision that is made across the top of the skull from ear to ear. We either place the incision in or slightly in front of the hairline, depending on the individual needs of our patient. Because both scalp advancement and forehead feminization require the same incision in or in front of the hairline, these procedures are generally completed together. Both procedures (scalp advancement and forehead feminization) are inpatient surgeries performed under general anesthesia with an overnight hospital stay.

TYPE I AND TYPE II FOREHEAD SKELETAL STRUCTURES

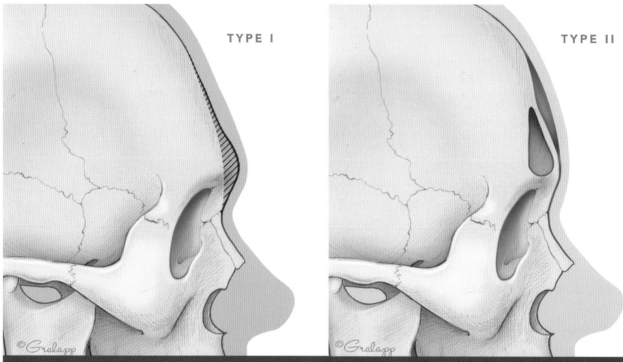

TYPE I

TYPE II

Illustrations depicting the difference between a Type I and a Type II forehead skeletal structure. Type I shows no frontal sinus. Type II shows concavity filled in.

Type I Procedure

Individuals who undergo a Type I procedure usually don't have as severe an issue with their foreheads as other transfeminine patients. During Dr. Ousterhout's time in practice, only 9 percent of transfeminine forehead patients, or eighty-five individuals, have needed this type of forehead correction. We are now finding that the number of true Type I foreheads is decreasing for reasons we do not totally understand. We have found that only 3 percent of cases can be successfully managed using burring alone.

The Type I procedure is designed for those who had no frontal sinuses or had a very small frontal sinus and/or a very thick anterior frontal sinus wall (thirty-two of the eighty-five patients). The Type I approach consists of burring away the excess forehead bone and developing a desired female contour without entering the frontal sinus, if it exists. Although it is the easiest of our four forehead approaches, it must be accomplished in the presence of the thin underlying frontal sinus, if there is one. In that case, if it is burred down to be too thin, then it is vulnerable to trauma or injury.

Type II Procedure

This operation is designed for patients with normal sinuses and a normal, desirable female forehead protrusion with standard bossing and the concavity above it. A small number (only 8 percent) of our transfeminine forehead procedures are suitable for a Type II approach because the projection is already where we want it. Again, this type of operation seems to

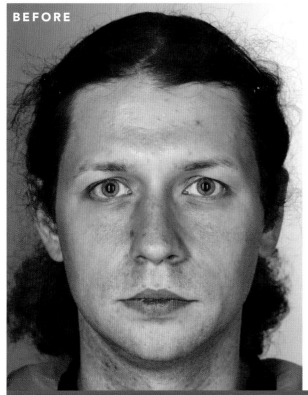
BEFORE

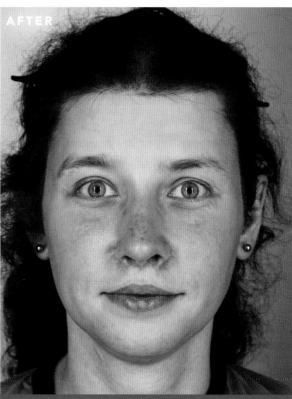
AFTER

Initially this patient had a thyroid cartilage reduction (Adam's apple reduction), and then returned for surgery to feminize her forehead, a rhinoplasty and an upper lip lift, and fat grafting (fat injections).

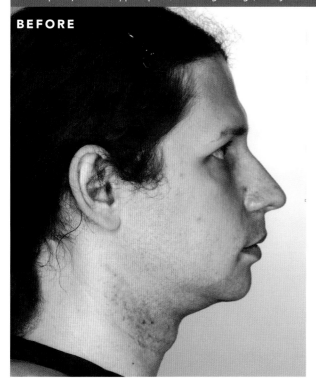
BEFORE

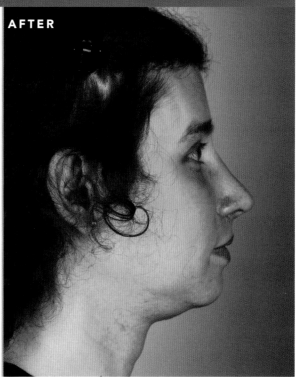
AFTER

be dwindling in terms of actual numbers. We see this approximately one or two times for every fifty cases, making the percentage approximately 2 to 4 percent of forehead feminizations.

Only the concavity needs to be addressed in a Type II approach. Even though we are not doing significant bone contouring with this technique, we reduce some of the bossing above and to the side of the brow as well as any hooding. We leave the frontal sinuses alone, but we fill the concave area above the bossing with hydroxyapatite bone cement that allows a near perfect contour to correct the concavity. This technique is particularly useful in Asian individuals who need or want only minimal changes to their forehead protrusion for feminization.

Dr. Ousterhout formerly used methyl methacrylate exclusively for forehead augmentation. There are some other materials now available that have some advantages over methyl methacrylate.

Type III Procedure

A Type III approach is used for the frontal sinus, which appears in 95 percent of all people, and for the masculine projection of the forehead. This projection appears in nearly every male and extends well beyond any female projection. The great majority, some 90 percent, of our forehead feminizations are Type III operations. We have performed Type III operations on more than 1,800 transfeminine patients and many other non-transgender individuals as well.

During this procedure, we remove the anterior or frontal sinus bone and contour the entire forehead into a more feminine shape. The excised bone is then configured to fit back into and cover the hole created by cutting out part of the frontal sinus wall. In some cases, it may be necessary to harvest and use a cranial bone graft to completely close the opening created by removing part of the frontal sinus bone. This generally occurs if a patient has large sinuses and/or a very thin or curved frontal sinus wall.

For this correction, there is no other option in terms of suitable materials. Using a rib or hip (*iliac crest*) bone graft would not only require another incision, but it would produce an inadequate result. Why? The only successful way to cover the anterior frontal sinus wall is to use a similar material or bone. Because both rib and hip bones are different types of bones than the skull, they would produce an inadequate result. That leaves a cranial bone graft as the only plausible solution. Even bone substitutes or materials, such as hydroxyapatite, do not work and should not be tried.

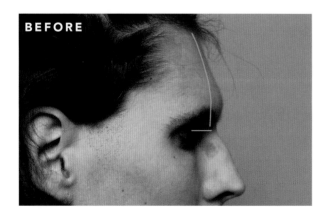

BEFORE

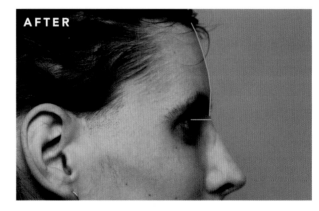

AFTER

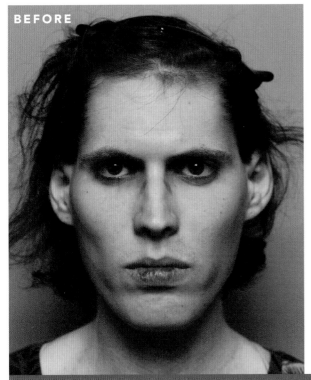

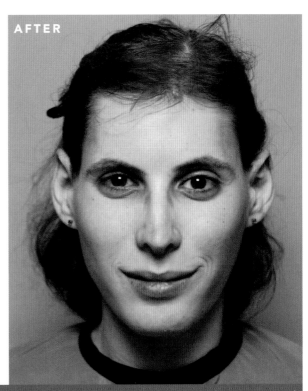

Before and after facial feminization surgery. Procedures included: forehead contouring Type III, scalp advancement (hairline lowering), brow lift, rhinoplasty, genioplasty (chin reshaping using osteotomies), and jaw tapering (feminizing or reducing the size of the jaw).

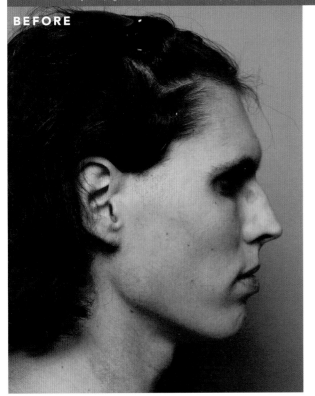

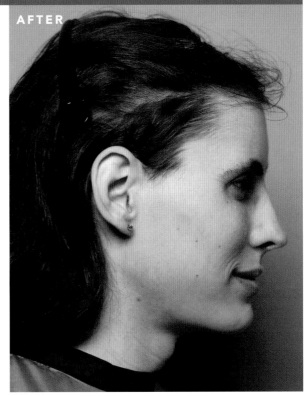

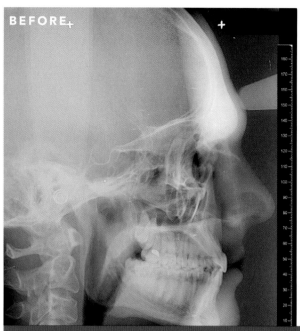 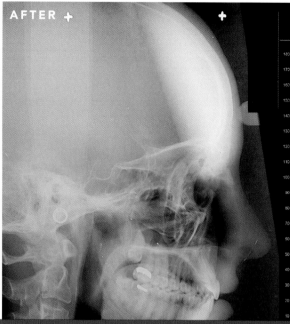

Before and after forehead feminization. This individual had no frontal sinus necessitating a Type I reconstruction.

In any case, there is no problem in addressing the frontal sinuses in this procedure. We simply reconstruct the anterior wall, anchoring the bone by wiring it in place with very fine surgical wire. Occasionally, we will use some very thin titanium plates and miniature screws.

Some people have asked us why we do not routinely use more modern plates and screws to stabilize the forehead. We do occasionally use several plates and screws while working on an unusual Type III forehead; however, as a patient continues to take estrogen medications, the skin tends to become thinner and occasionally the plates and screws may be felt.

Still, very thin plates and small screws are commonly used in cranial surgeries, including those on the forehead. They work very well. Normally, if used properly, they cannot be felt through the skin.

If they can be felt, we have heard other surgeons say that they deal with this by burring off the top of the plate and screw. Yet, this would make subsequent removal of the screws and plates nearly impossible. We also find burring a poor way to mitigate the problem. If one measures the diameter of twisted wire, it is 200 microns thick. For comparison, that is about the thickness of a typical sheet of paper. When one measures the thickness of commercially available plates and screws, they are 350 microns thick.

Using modern plates and screws is easier for the surgeon and requires less surgical skill compared to fixation with very fine surgical wire. Using the fine wire fixation technique also takes a bit longer. We typically use the fine wire technique because it gives a better overall result, even though it takes longer in the operating room. Using the wire fixation method allows one to get a tighter fit of the mating bone surfaces.

There are some circumstances in which we may use a combination of both methods. Ultimately, we wire the bone and sinuses so that

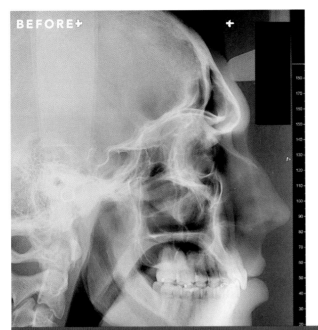 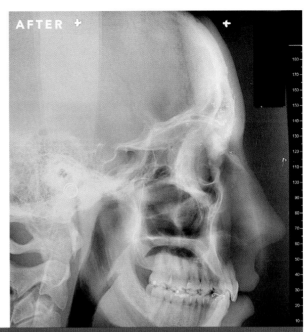

This patient has a very large frontal sinus requiring a Type III contouring procedure. The wires holding the bone graft in place are apparent in the postsurgical scan. The chin, jawline, and angle of the jaw were also reduced considerably.

they are not only intact and secure, but also function properly after surgery. There is an old surgical adage that stainless steel and titanium should not be used together. We have not found this to be a problem as long as the two metals are not actually touching one another.

We routinely turn to the Type III procedure, because neither of us can put the anterior frontal sinus wall back into a desirable position with any other method. Given what we can accomplish with this procedure, it is a must for achieving a desired female contour and the best aesthetic result. Although this is the most time-consuming of the forehead surgical approaches, the results are stellar.

One last comment regarding the Type III forehead. Often, patients ask for a reconstruction of their forehead that does not involve any foreign material. Some surgeons have suggested to people that this method is possible, and they

have attempted surgeries in this manner. This method is not recommended. A core tenet of craniofacial surgery is rigid fixation of bone segments. Rigid fixation allows the bones to heal at their boundaries. The sinus is a dynamic cavity that undergoes changes in pressure as you breathe, and that micro-motion must be essentially eliminated during the time of healing; otherwise, the bone graft will, eventually, resorb and you will be left with a defect or hole in your frontal sinus which will require a second operation to correct.

Type IV Procedure

We opt for a Type IV approach when a forehead is too narrow or too far back to realize a desirable contour using one of the three previous surgeries described. In the nine Type IV cases Dr. Deschamps-Braly has completed to date, he built up or augmented the entire forehead, using methyl methacrylate, the medical polymer or

SURGICAL STEPS INVOLVED IN A TYPE III FOREHEAD FEMINIZATION

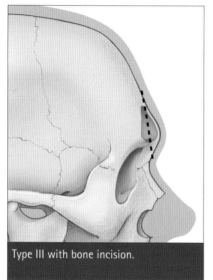

Type III with bone incision.

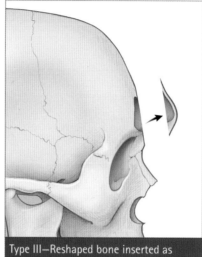

Type III—Reshaped bone inserted as shown below.

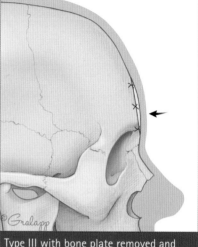

Type III with bone plate removed and reshaped.

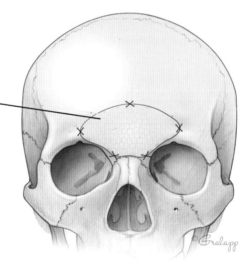

Surgically reshaped bone plate installed and secured.

plastic resin that you might know commercially as Lucite. We have used some other materials successfully and feel that methyl methacrylate is a great material. However, it may not be the only good material that is now available.

The advantage of methyl methacrylate is that it is easy for a surgeon to use. We simply mix and apply the material directly to the site, molding it into the correct forehead configuration before it hardens. The methyl methacrylate can then be sculpted with rotating burrs to a final desired contour. If we need to add more material, we can do it easily.

Methyl methacrylate works extremely well in feminizing these two forehead areas: Type II and IV. The use of this material in other areas is subject to some controversy, but that concern is unwarranted when used for feminizing foreheads. The material is not only very effective, but also very safe.

There are also other materials that have as much promise as methyl methacrylate and are much easier to use. Newer materials, including polymer hydroxyapatites, actually adhere to the bone, making fixation of the implant unimportant. They are composed of alternative isomers that the body recognizes as normal bone. However, they cannot be resorbed by your body.

Nasal Radix Needs Attention

Feminizing the forehead in patients who need Type I, II, or III surgery involves another consideration: how the forehead and nose intersect at the *radix*, the bony area between the eyes at the top of the nose. Women and men differ not only in the prominence of the forehead, but also in the way the nose juts onto the face at the radix. The prominence of the radix is more gradual in females and more angular in males. What do we mean by angular? The chiseled profile of Dick Tracy is only an exaggerated cartoon, but as a male, you probably have a variation of his look.

To create a smooth, acceptable transition, rather than an abrupt, unacceptable juncture between the forehead and nose, we feminize the forehead first before bringing the nose in line at the radix. In most cases, the front or anterior of the forehead must be moved behind the front or anterior of the radix. Properly reducing the radix after such contouring ensures a normal-looking nose along with a nose-to-forehead junction that slopes gently.

Because the radix may have to be set back as much as 8 or 9 mm behind the preoperative position of the nose, your surgeon cannot complete the repositioning safely with a standard rhinoplasty, which is nose reshaping. Why? Because it risks creating a *fistula*, an abnormal passageway into the frontal sinus, by contouring the nose from below, which is the usual approach with rhinoplasty. In our experience, working from above, while completing appropriate forehead contouring, is the only way to set the radix back safely and effectively.

So, we tell patients it is okay to do a rhinoplasty without a forehead feminization. But if you're going to feminize your forehead, you almost always need to deal with the nose at the same time to prevent a nasal deformity. Only in rare cases would you leave the nose alone. In our last 850 cases, we felt it was acceptable to leave the nose alone in just ten patients. Essentially, only 1 percent of noses do not need modification at the time of forehead feminization.

If you decide after a rhinoplasty that you want to feminize your forehead, the surgery will involve your nose again. The goal is to achieve the right relationship between the two features. We'll discuss this further in chapter 7.

Importance of Forehead Measurements

For more than twenty-five years, we have measured the distance the forehead extends forward beyond the eyes in both transfeminine transgender and other patients. These calibrations (from more than 2,000 transfeminine patients alone) have proven very valuable. They have confirmed the marked differences between the sexes and have guided our surgical decision making and planning for every forehead feminization.

The normal range for forehead protrusion in men is on average higher than the normal range in women. In fact, the lowest measurements in males are generally higher than the highest measurements in females. An even more important consideration for feminization is that the forehead measurements of attractive females are almost always lower than the lowest normal

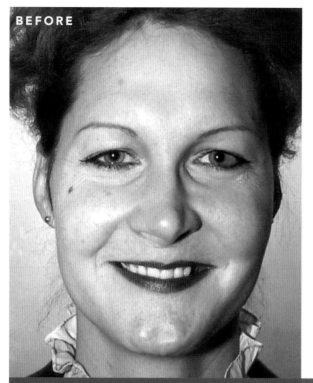

BEFORE

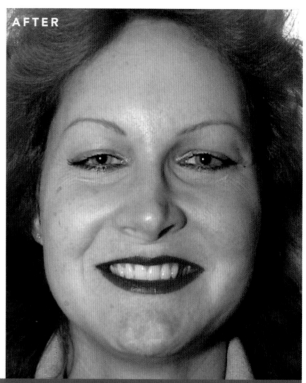

AFTER

Photos on the left are prior to Type II forehead feminization. Photos on the right are after forehead contouring. No other FFS procedures were performed.

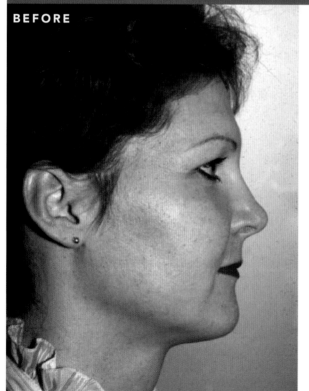

BEFORE

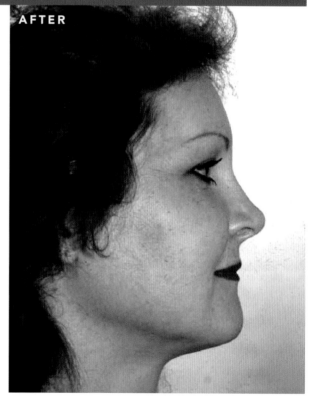

AFTER

measurement for their gender. We first discovered this in one of our patients and have since confirmed it in many other attractive females.

When we first started forehead feminizations thirty-five years ago, we used the average female measurement as our end point. Several years afterward, however, one patient, whom we had already feminized to an "average" forehead position, came back with photographs of many models whose profiles she admired.

We couldn't measure the foreheads on the models' pictures, but it was obvious that their protrusion was much less than what we had been using as the desired end point of our surgeries. Our patient asked us if we could redo her forehead, so we contoured her prominence with a Type III procedure to reflect the position in the photos of the models. It worked beautifully. The new method made a significant difference in the final result. She was much prettier after her second procedure than after her first surgery.

After that experience, we realized that to give our transfeminine patients the most attractive look possible, we had to do more than just rely on "average" female calibrations to remodel their foreheads. We could produce better results by decreasing the protrusion even farther than the average in most women. Since that time, we've dramatically changed our forehead feminizations, giving our transfeminine patients a prettier prominence than in the past.

We have also used these calibrations many times in men who just want a more masculine forehead. In other cases, we've used the measurements for men whose foreheads are so prominent, often because of very large frontal sinuses, that they look sinister. Since performing the first such operation ever on a patient with this problem in

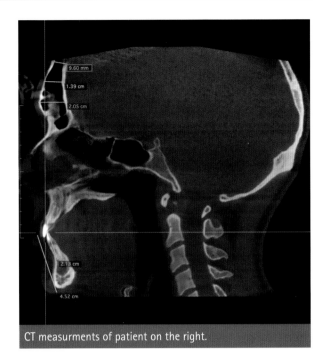

CT measurments of patient on the right.

1982, we have done more than 2,300 such Type III procedures on both sexes.

We also note that more is not always better. It is true that overcorrecting a forehead will create beautiful features. Yet, there are some people, particularly those who have very projected radixes, for whom the skin between their eyes will not contract and conform, leading to some excessive skin there. Patients will suggest that their eyes look different somehow. We have found that careful consideration of the patient's skin quality and projection is necessary when preparing for surgery to minimize the risk of this happening.

Finding the Right Surgeon

Over the years, it has become obvious to us, from meeting many transfeminine individuals other than our patients, that a number of facial feminization surgeons do not understand the measurements regarding forehead projection and the associated results of different surgical

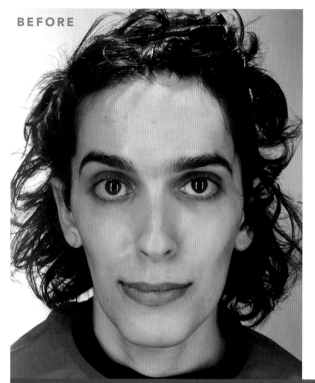

BEFORE

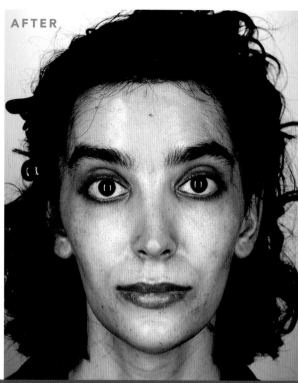

AFTER

FFS procedures: Type III forehead contouring, scalp advancement, brow lift, rhinoplasty, and chin reshaping to shorten and narrow the chin.

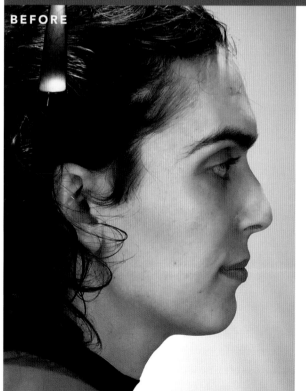

BEFORE

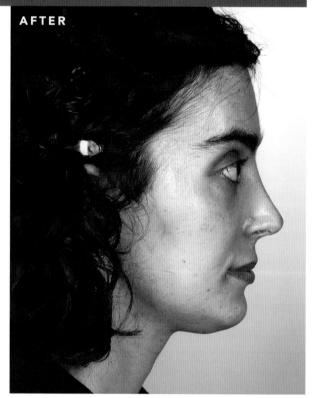

AFTER

approaches. Some surgeons do not know how to address the unique forehead challenges presented by each patient. A well-meaning surgeon, for instance, may try to achieve a feminized forehead in someone with significant frontal sinus and forehead prominence by simply doing a small, bony reduction on the brows. But that patient may really need orbital rim setback, contouring, and other procedures. Failing to use the appropriate surgical approach will lead to disappointment for the patient in their final appearance after healing from the surgery.

Extensive experience in both craniofacial surgery and the varied approaches described in this book, are essential to successfully feminize the forehead. On more than one occasion, each of us has been extremely grateful that we were trained as craniofacial surgeons because we could handle the unexpected events that surfaced during surgery. For example, one transfeminine patient had a small, previously unknown *encephalocele,* an abnormal sac-like protrusion of the brain appearing in her frontal sinus. We easily repaired the encephalocele and grafted bone in the area. Another patient injured her mid-forehead and upper nose when her car collided with a backhoe just ten days after her initial surgery, causing multiple fractures. She returned immediately to San Francisco, and we repaired the problem by placing cranial bone grafts. Thankfully, she recovered without deformity.

If you are pursuing a forehead feminization, make sure your surgeon understands the measurable differences between male and female foreheads and can adjust for them with an approach that fits your features and needs. You want a plastic surgeon who is also qualified as a craniofacial surgeon in order to have a surgeon who is competent to handle any surprises that will, inevitably over time, come a long way.

Correcting Previous Surgeries

Currently, approximately 15 percent of the FFS patients we see in our office seek secondary surgeries, most often on the forehead. This percentage is nearly twice the percentage of people who sought secondary surgeries a decade ago. These patients come not only from the United States, but also from Europe, South America, Latin America, the Middle East, and Asia.

The cause of these secondary operations is usually an inadequate primary forehead reduction that was never adequately feminized in the first place. The previous surgeon, using either a direct vision or endoscopic approach, may only have burred away the bone as best as possible given the limitations of the surgeon's philosophy and approach to this surgery. Often, these are done when a more extensive procedure (usually Type III) is actually needed. The result of the initial inadequate surgery is often far too much forehead projection, requiring a second surgery for a result that is truly satisfactory to these patients.

In some instances, the previous surgeon stopped short of completing the procedure, because the surgeon had entered the frontal sinus by shaving the bone. If that bone is burred to near paper thinness, it may be too weak to withstand minor trauma to the face. In addition, if the thinness from improper contouring results in bony holes, blowing one's nose can then cause the overlying skin to inflate or bulge forward.

In our experience, the original surgeons in these situations have done nothing to close any bony holes that might have occurred with this inappropriate surgical approach. In some instances, the surgeons have filled the defect with a silicone-like material. By the time the patient sees us, there is already a significant infection in the frontal sinus. In other cases, the doctor has tried the Type III procedure, but the forehead still projected too far forward and was irregular in contour.

One additional note on secondary surgeries: Some surgeons who do forehead contouring don't believe a Type III procedure can be redone. This is not true. We have never seen any case that we could not redo. These situations usually require a *cranial bone graft* (harvesting bone from the skull for transplant to the forehead). On the surface, using such a graft may seem like a big issue, but cranial bone implants are not dangerous. They are ideal for properly reconstructing the sinus. Whatever the challenge left by your first surgery, the approach for a secondary operation is exactly the same as for a primary procedure—but done correctly.

After Your Forehead Feminization Surgery

Regardless of which forehead approach your surgeon uses, there is basically no difference in the postoperative pain, swelling, or recovery time you'll experience with this surgery. Currently, our patients typically spend only one night in the hospital and then leave the hospital the day after surgery. Whether you are undergoing this procedure alone, or with scalp advancement, you'll need to pay attention to the same guidelines.

Recovery and Follow-up Care

After forehead feminization, you'll leave the operating room with stitches in the pre-hairline area of your forehead and staples in your scalp. Pain or discomfort can be addressed easily with medication, whereas any swelling and bruising

you experience around the eyes usually recedes within ten to twelve days. If you work at home you can return to work that week, but most individuals return to their daily activities in two weeks. At the same time, you should not do anything for two weeks that would cause you to sweat or raise your blood pressure or pulse.

Side Effects and Potential Complications

As with scalp advancement, forehead feminization is usually a well-tolerated surgery. The results can be dramatic, offering patients a powerful psychological pick-me-up. Most patients have no problem with the side effects that come with this operation because they are largely temporary. Although recovery should be relatively event free, be aware of the following potential issues.

Infection from Methyl Methacrylate after Forehead Surgery

The primary infection concern with forehead feminization involves methyl methacrylate that is sometimes used during Type II and Type IV forehead surgeries to round the contours of the forehead. If you develop an infection from contouring with this material, you would most likely need to have your implant removed. However, we have never lost one of these implants in an FFS patient.

It is very difficult to treat an infection around any implant, be it chin, breast, hip, knee, or other prosthesis. It is particularly difficult next to the bone. We have used methyl methacrylate in hundreds of patients. In two patients (not FFS patients) that involved rather unusual circumstances, Dr. Ousterhout had to remove methyl methacrylate implants.

One patient who required removal of methyl methacrylate implant, had his forehead reconstructed for a major congenital craniofacial deformity. Seven years later, a car hit him as he was walking across a freeway. This young man's head went through the windshield. Radiographs showed no skull fractures. However, about seven months after the accident, pus started draining from his left temple.

This patient returned to San Francisco where we removed the implant and found a previously unknown fracture from the accident of the anterior wall of the frontal sinus—the obvious source of the pus and bacteria. We repaired the fracture, sterilized the implant, and replaced it seven months later. It has been there for seventeen years with no problems. The second of these two patients had undergone major post-cancer skull reconstruction with methyl methacrylate. A few years later, he had a heart transplant. Unfortunately, his chest incision from that surgery became infected. The bacteria then affected the earlier forehead implant, which had to be removed.

Other Forehead-Related Infections

The small number of infections we have encountered with our forehead feminization patients have been caused by existing frontal sinus disease. In some cases, the preexisting frontal sinus disease was uncovered during surgery. This has occurred in about 10 percent of individuals undergoing Type III procedures. Please do not let that one-in-ten percentage scare you. It turned out that finding these problems was actually a good thing. In two cases, infection-related pus appeared ready to break through the back of the frontal sinus and into the front lobes of the brain.

The simple reality is that their elective FFS forehead surgery resulted in timely diagnoses of their underlying infections. These patients were facing dire, even possibly fatal, infections. So, correcting the forehead drainage system during their forehead feminization surgery may actually have saved their lives.

In the other individuals with forehead-related infections, the condition was not nearly so severe, but still was abnormal. These patients often had significant sinus disease, as shown by the thick, gelatinous, deep yellow mucous lining of the sinus. The infection was probably caused by a partial obstruction, most likely from a previous nasal injury or allergy. In some cases, there were polyps in the sinus cavity, which is not uncommon in patients with allergies.

When only one *(unilateral)* side of the sinus is infected, it is treated rather easily by draining the cavity into the opposite side. When both sides *(bilateral)* are involved, an alternate draining system is created by drilling into the ethmoid air cells, a collection of thin-walled cavities between the nose and the eyes. Drainage can occur through these cavities.

In all the sinus infections related to obstruction that we have treated, CT scans were taken of the patients' frontal sinuses about a month after surgery. We could then check for fluid that might signal the continuing presence of an obstruction. In each case, not only was there no fluid, but the mucosa also had returned to normal, suggesting that the problem had been corrected. Obviously, this surgery had a positive effect on our patients' health, beyond just forehead feminization.

Sinus Headaches

A number of patients complain before surgery of frontal sinus headaches. Although we haven't tracked the statistics, we are confident we have had more than one hundred patients

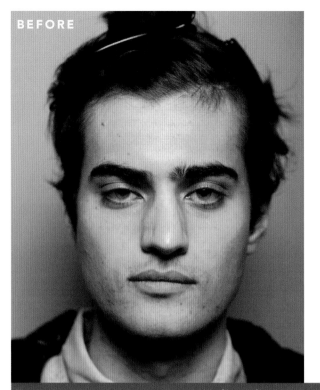
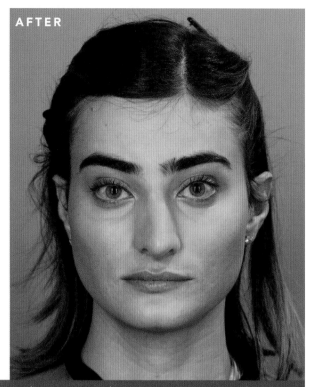

This patient underwent forehead contouring (Type III), scalp advancement (hairline lowering), chin, and jaw feminization (chin being cut, narrowed, and reduced in height), thyroid cartilage reduction (trach shave or Adam's apple shave), and pan facial fat grafting (fat injections to the face).

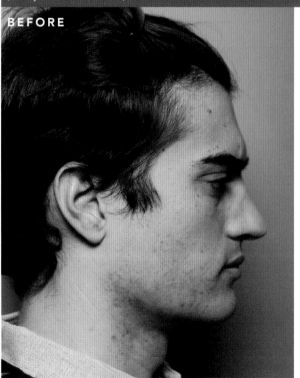
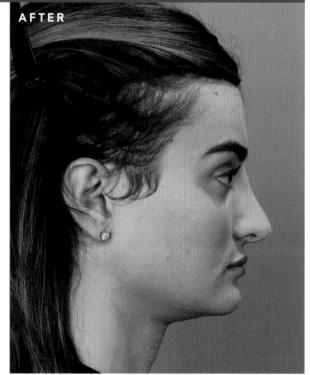

with such complaints. Yet, we have only found frontal sinus disease that might explain the headaches—probably due to allergies—in two of these patients. The cause of the headaches in the other ninety-eight patients remains a mystery.

Numbness

Some surgeons warn about scalp and forehead numbness following the coronal incision, yet in fact, it is often not a problem. The reassuring news is that any loss of feeling is usually only temporary and isn't a reason to avoid this part of facial feminization. You should consider the following, however, regarding loss of sensation.

To make the initial incision across the top of the head for scalp advancement and/or forehead feminization, your surgeon must cut the superior orbital nerve. This nerve reaches across the forehead to the back of the ears. The only way to avoid tampering with the superior orbital nerve is with an endoscopic technique, in which the surgeon uses special fiber-optic instruments inserted through a keyhole incision to move the tissue.

Even though your surgeon may recommend this approach as a less invasive way to feminize your forehead, and avoid that nerve, it does not allow for satisfactory forehead contouring or scalp advancement. An endoscopic approach may reduce the amount of numbness you feel after surgery, but even with this technique, a significant percentage of patients still experience temporary or permanent loss of scalp sensation. The bottom line is that the forehead cannot be properly feminized with an endoscopic approach.

As to any loss of feeling behind your incision, the numbness can affect a very small area or may be as large as your fist. Because the length of the superior orbital nerve varies tremendously, some patients will experience little or no numbness at all. In about 98 percent of individuals who do have lack of sensation after surgery, feeling comes back in about twelve to eighteen months. On rare occasions, it will take between two to two and a half years.

In 1 to 2 percent of patients, feeling may not return at all. Like any other numbness that occurs after surgery or from a significant laceration or cut, patients soon forget the numbness. It is rarely, if ever, a long-term issue. So, concern about loss of sensation in your forehead or scalp for a short time postoperatively should not cause you to avoid the operation.

Forehead Paralysis

None of our patients have suffered forehead paralysis from forehead feminization. The branches of the seventh cranial or facial nerve that reach into the forehead, lie in the soft tissue, where they stimulate the forehead muscles; these muscles allow one to show expressions such as frowning and showing surprise. Because forehead surgery is completed at the bony level, these nerves are not typically subject to injury.

Bone Loss

One of the most amazing things about forehead feminization, is that there is no bone loss with a Type III procedure, because it involves cranial bone grafting to cover the anterior frontal sinus wall. Ideally, bone should be transferred as a vascularized graft, meaning that its blood supply remains completely intact. When the bone is removed during this procedure, it is taken away from its blood supply. Yet, that supply is eventually restored to the superficial side when the bone is repositioned and wired into place. It is not immediately restored, however, on the sinus side. Classically, bone grafts do very poorly without a blood supply, but in a Type III procedure, the bone does extremely well.

In fact, to the best of our knowledge, we have never lost even one bone graft with a Type III procedure. To ensure there is no bone loss, grafts taken from the cranium are a must if any bone grafting is needed for anterior frontal sinus closure. In addition, the bone graft must be rigidly fixated with either wire or thin plates and tiny screws to avoid resorption of the graft.

Outcome of Surgery

The results of our forehead contouring surgeries have been most successful. Our patients are usually ecstatic over their new profiles. By going beyond the necessary bone contouring, we've been able to reduce the hooding, bossing, and projection in ways unique to each person. In many cases, the changes accomplished by these forehead techniques are remarkable. Contouring the skeletal orbits around the eyes, for instance, opens the area up so much that transfeminine patients no longer have to hide their masculine foreheads behind bangs. They can sweep their hair back, exposing a feminized profile and an open-eyed look. With the proper approach, forehead feminization can dramatically impact a patient's appearance and happiness.

Commonly Asked Questions

A Type III forehead contouring sounds pretty scary. Do I have reason to be afraid? No. This should not be a scary surgery. Consider the source if you have heard these kinds of concerns from other transgender patients who have elected not to have the procedure or from surgeons who do not know how to perform the surgery correctly. Type III forehead feminization is no more painful than other procedures.

It generally does not take longer to heal or cause more bruising than other feminization operations. If you have a typical masculine forehead (which you probably do), with a normal frontal sinus and a normal thin anterior or frontal sinus bone, contouring alone will not achieve the desired result. You have no choice but to undergo a Type III procedure if you want an aesthetically pleasing outcome.

Can you do the procedure under local anesthesia? Technically, yes one could, but there are practical reasons why this is a poor idea. We don't recommend this type of anesthesia for our patients.

My doctor says I do not need a Type III procedure. What do you think? If a lateral cephalogram was not ordered, your surgeon has no idea of your needs. If your doctor has ordered the test, however, make sure you see your skull radiograph. Ask your doctor to point out your frontal sinus, its contour, and the thickness of the anterior wall bone. Then ask how that surgeon intends to correct your problem.

My friends say my forehead looks great. Do I need surgery? You should consider whether there is some question in your mind about how feminine you really appear. Does your forehead look great because it really is a feminine forehead? Or does it look good because you are covering it with bangs? Friends often give the worst advice. Depending on the friend and their particular biases, you may receive a lot of advice that is not based on reality.

Often, acquaintances may criticize your choice to have surgery, or the result after the surgery, simply because they are envious. Again, friends and loved ones very rarely give unbiased or knowledgeable advice about changing your appearance. If you have questions, do not just guess at the answers. Please schedule a consultation. Yes, we charge a fee for a consultation, but it will be money well spent. With a consultation and the appropriate cephalogram, we can give you a definitive evaluation of your individual situation.

I am sixty-six years old. Is it too late for me to have this forehead surgery? No. We do not think there is an age limit, as long as you are healthy enough for the surgery. We have performed the procedure on many patients in their sixties, even two in their seventies. They all did well.

I am nineteen years old. Will my frontal sinus get larger in the next few years? It is possible if you are still growing, but if your height has not changed for the past year or two, your frontal sinus will not change size.

I need a Type III forehead procedure, but I also have to wear a helmet at work and when I ride my motorcycle. Can I wear either helmet right after surgery? What are my limitations? As with broken limbs and other types of bone healing, you probably need extended time to heal completely before you may wear rigid headgear that rests on your forehead.

This usually is not an issue for most people, but if you must wear a helmet for work or motorcycle riding, you should probably avoid wearing the helmet for six to seven weeks to allow the forehead to heal well. Otherwise, you risk causing a deformity. We had one patient who jousted in full armor. Certainly, in these cases, we recommend extended time without wearing the headgear.

Why are you so adamant about the training of doctors who perform forehead surgery? There are four different operations (Type I, Type II, Type III, and Type IV) that a surgeon can do to feminize the forehead. Only Type I, which

represents 9 percent of all cases, is a relatively simple contouring procedure. That doesn't mean, however, that all surgeons do it well. A surgeon might be able to perform a Type I forehead procedure properly with an endoscope in the mid-forehead. Yet, this approach is not safe, especially when eliminating lateral hooding.

The other procedures are even more complex and require the expertise of a specialist trained in craniofacial surgery to perform them safely with consistent good results. Physicians don't learn these kinds of techniques while training as a plastic surgeon or as an *ear, nose, and throat (ENT)* resident. No matter how good these specialists are in their respective disciplines, their training is not sufficient to handle either the procedure or the types of complications that can occur with it.

For instance, in approximately 70 percent of our secondary forehead surgeries, the patient has required a cranial bone graft. This is not routine surgery, especially for a surgeon who is not trained in craniofacial surgery. Finally, we have found significant preexisting disease in the frontal sinus in more than 10 percent of our Type III patients. Neither we nor the patients knew about these conditions prior to surgery. In two cases, the infections were potentially life-threatening. Yet, we knew what to do because we have each been trained as craniofacial surgeons and have each seen these conditions before.

As you can gather from these examples (and there are many more), all of these situations must be handled on the spot, not left for another time or another specialist. Applying the proper treatment requires experience over many years. We strongly believe that only someone formally trained in craniofacial surgery is fully competent to perform these forehead feminization procedures and is able to deal with any ensuing complications or health issues. Please do not ignore this caution, because to do so, puts you at risk.

Does a Type III procedure cost more than a Type I procedure? Yes. Depending upon the size of your sinus and the thickness of the bone, a Type III procedure may take one to two hours longer than a Type I surgery. Charges for the anesthesiologist and the hospital operating room are calculated in fifteen-minute segments. Because this surgery is longer than a Type I operation, you will accumulate a few more segments, which will add to the cost. In addition, your plastic surgeon is likely to charge more for longer procedures than shorter ones.

A Final Note

Many transfeminine individuals think they do not need forehead contouring because they can pass without it. They'll just let their bangs camouflage the bossing and hooding; they may also let bangs cover a hairline that may be receding or brows that are characteristically low and straight. By contrast, women's hairlines tend to be arch-shaped and closer to their eyebrows, which tend to curve above the orbital rims. Without feminization, your forehead will always be a giveaway to your birth gender. But with the right approach, you should no longer have to worry about "just passing" as a woman.

5

Temporal Fossa Augmentation

THE *TEMPORAL FOSSA* IS THE shallow depression of your skull just to the side of your eyes, above your cheekbones. You know it as your temple. Created by an underlying pair of cranial or temporal bones, it houses the temporalis muscle, one of the strong muscles necessary for chewing. If you take away the muscle, you are left with a space called the *temporal fossa*.

Normally, this indentation is a discreet hollow just below and behind your forehead. But if the depression is so pronounced that it makes you look sickly or gaunt, you may want your surgeon to fill it in. Augmenting a temporal fossa depression isn't a necessary step in feminizing your face, but it will add immensely to a healthy, feminized look.

Assessing the Temporal Fossa

There is no difference between the sexes when it comes to having an exaggerated temporal fossa depression. A deeply concave or inwardly curved space usually has nothing to do with gender. Whether you have male or female genetics, a pronounced hollow, just behind your lateral orbital rims—or the bony ridges to the side of your eyes—will have a significant effect on your facial aesthetics. This hollow can make you appear to be starving when you are actually well fed.

Although most people don't have a temporal fossa depression that merits attention, it is not an uncommon occurrence. The degree and precise location, however, can be variable. Also, the depression isn't necessarily symmetrical—the same on both sides. When it does exist, augmenting the space can offer many aesthetic benefits. Improving the contour can create a more appealing look.

Undergoing Temporal Fossa Depression Surgery

The temporal fossa can be treated in four ways: using preformed implants, fat injections, the medical plastic resin methyl methacrylate, or other bone cements. Treatment of the temporal fossa usually takes place along with other forehead-recontouring procedures. The temporal fossa depression portion of the surgery takes about an hour. As you will learn shortly, the methyl methacrylate approach involves lifting muscle from the bone, so the surgery must be performed under general anesthesia.

Preformed Implant Approach

Your surgeon may suggest preformed implants to augment your temporal fossa, but we are not a fan of them. The standard choice is the MEDPOR surgical implant, which is created from a biomaterial called *linear high-density polyethylene,* or *PEEK (Poly-Ether-Ether-Ketone).* There may be other models available as well. Custom-made implants are now possible, based on CT scans, computer-aided (CAD/CAM) milling, or 3-D printing technology.

Temporal fossa depressions differ in size, shape, and even location from person to person. Preformed implants, by their very nature, cannot be easily modified to deal with the many variations we see in patients. This is not a one-size-or-shape-fits-all procedure. As such, we don't believe surgeons can do a proper augmentation with this medium.

Fat Grafting Approach

Fat grafting (also called *fat injection*) is a proven, well-accepted augmentation method frequently used for various parts of the body. We prefer extensive fat grafting for temporal fossa treatment.

We take fat from the inner thigh because the fat there tends to be less stringy and has less fibrous material. It also has a greater number of stem cells than in other areas of the body. This can improve the quality of skin after injection. For more on fat grafting, see chapter 6 on cheek contouring.

After harvesting the fat, it is purified and then injected with 1-cc syringes using 0.9 mm cannulas (tubes). To inject the fat, we only release about one-twentieth of 1 cc of fat. Thus, we might pass

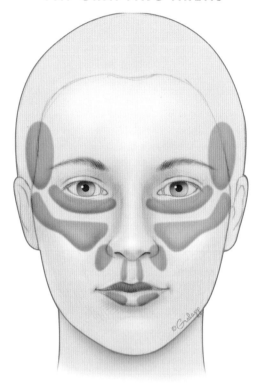

FAT GRAFTING AREAS

Illustration shows the areas where fat grafting is most commonly used to fill in "sunken" areas.

the needle through the tissue twenty or thirty times before we go through one syringe of material. Injecting the fat in small, very fine amounts provides the best chance of its survival after it is placed.

We have seen the occasional problem with both fat grafting and methyl methacrylate approaches. Fat grafting is a little less predictable; however, the material is natural. Occasionally, the procedure may need to be performed twice to obtain a great result. In our experience, it rarely causes lumpiness.

Best of all, there are rarely serious complications with this procedure. Because the fat is *autologous* (obtained from your own body), there is no inflammatory response after injection.

Thus, there is a reduced risk for side effects after the procedure.

Yet fat grafting is a tissue graft like any other, and there can be some resorption or part of the graft may not survive. Most often, about 60 percent of the graft survives and the fraction that survives is permanent, safe, and natural.

Fat grafts include an abundance of stem cells. These cells act as natural repair and rejuvenation mechanisms in the body. Thus, they have the ability to improve skin texture, thickness, and elasticity after the fat is injected.

Methyl Methacrylate Approach

Methyl methacrylate is a material that is both compatible with human tissue and stable over time. So, it also offers a permanent solution to temporal fossa depressions. This acrylic or plastic resin offers versatility in many fields, including medicine. It is soft and moldable when mixed, but hard and fixed after it polymerizes, which takes only a few minutes.

Because methyl methacrylate is compatible with tissue, it can be injected into a space or placed safely in or on certain areas of the body to replace, remodel, or support lost and injured parts. This material is the cement used to stabilize hip prostheses. With pink coloring added to simulate the natural color of your gums, it has its most obvious use in dentures.

To accomplish this procedure, we expose the temporalis muscle and make short incisions in the back of it. Then, using an instrument called an *elevator,* we lift the muscle off the underlying bone to create a pocket in the area of the depression for the methyl methacrylate. In this maneuver, we raise only the area that we want to reshape, so that the results will look normal. After the pocket is ready, the methyl

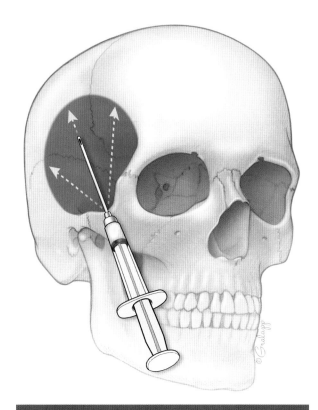

If the temple area is "sunken," a patient may benefit from a procedure that uses fat grafting to fill in the area.

methacrylate powder and liquid are mixed into white putty and placed into a syringe.

The material sets up almost immediately; therefore, we only have a few minutes or so of available work time. We quickly inject the methyl methacrylate into the pocket until the area is slightly overfilled. After the syringe is removed, we shape the material with our hands and fingertips and squeeze out any excess until we have an aesthetically pleasing result. Within ten to twelve minutes, the methyl methacrylate polymerizes and hardens into a rocklike substance with the weight and consistency of human bone. After everything is in place, the muscle incision is closed, followed at the appropriate

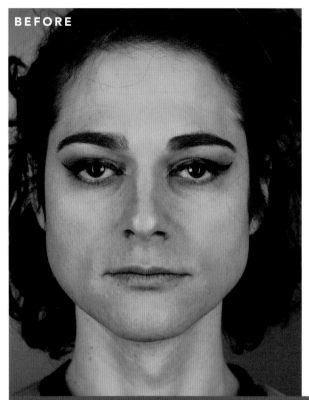

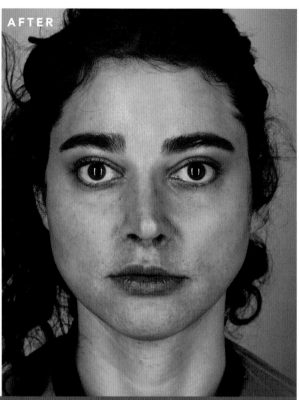

This patient underwent scalp advancement, forehead contouring Type III, brow lift, rhinoplasty, fat grafting, chin and jaw contouring, masseter reduction, upper lip lift, and thyroid cartilage reduction.

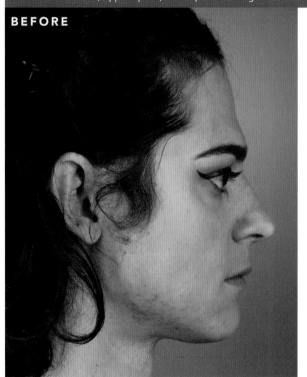

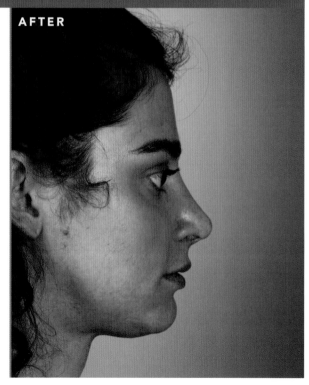

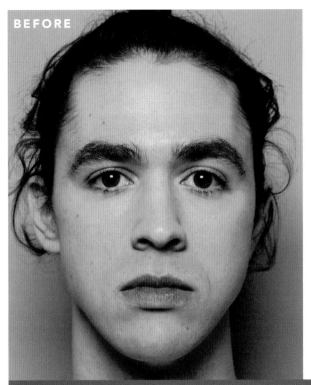

BEFORE

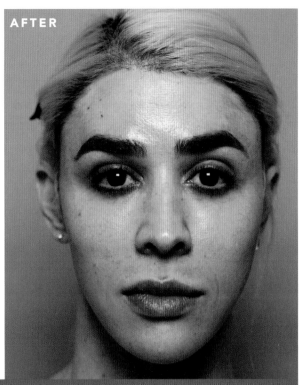

AFTER

Before and after fat grafting (injections) to the temples, cheeks, eye area, nasolabial fold, and upper lip. Other procedures: scalp advancement (hairline lowering), forehead Type III contouring, chin feminization (using bone cuts to reduce height and width), rhinoplasty (nose reshaping), jaw tapering, and thyroid cartilage reduction (Adam's apple reduction).

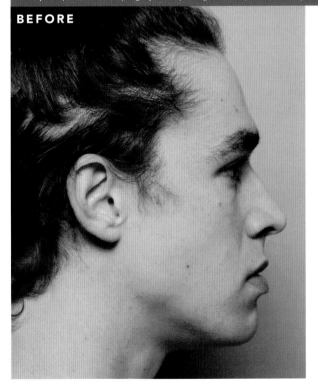

BEFORE

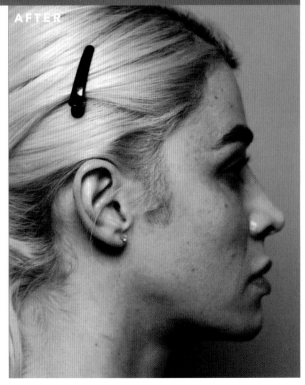

AFTER

time by closure of the scalp. The result is an improved, symmetrical temple contour.

Bone Cement

Bone cements are generally composed of either calcium phosphate or hydroxyapatite. There are a number of different ways that these cements are delivered from the manufacturer. Some are two-part mixtures that must be combined to form a hard cement; others are more difficult to work with due to various handling properties. The biggest issue with using a bone cement in this area is that it requires complete elevation of the temporalis muscle followed by resuspension. This often requires a significant amount of surgical work, and this approach has a high rate of complications. Therefore, our preferred technique is autologous fat grafting, mentioned earlier in this chapter.

After Your Temporal Fossa Surgery

If you are undergoing temporal fossa surgery, then you can look forward to a relatively quick, pain-free recovery. You will be placed on antibiotics to help prevent any complications such as infection. But you also will need to follow the additional instructions laid out by your surgeon. Many of them are common-sense steps to help you get the most out of this surgery.

Recovery and Follow-up Care

Patients undergoing temporal fossa surgery leave the operating room with a support garment wrapping the head. There are drains in place that are removed the morning after surgery. The scalp staples come out on the fourth to sixth day after surgery. The first hair wash should occur at the surgeon's office during your first postoperative visit. but you may shower the rest of your body the day after surgery. The instructions for returning to activity and work are the same as for other facial feminization surgeries. If you are working at home, you can return to your work duties the next day, although you probably want to make it a short day. If you do manual labor, you should not do heavy lifting for at least three weeks.

Side Effects and Potential Complications

Complications aren't usually associated with temporal fossa depression surgery. The small to moderate amount of swelling that occurs usually subsides within forty-eight to seventy-two hours. Pain is usually not an issue. Patients have not experienced *hematomas* (localized collections of blood), *seromas* (pockets of fluid that may develop after surgery), or infections with this procedure. It is very well tolerated in both the short and long term.

Outcome of Surgery

Not every transgender patient will need temporal fossa correction, but those who do, can anticipate a positive outcome. Dr. Ousterhout has performed this surgery in twenty-one transgender patients. Dr. Deschamps-Braly has used fat grafts for the temples in more than 400 patients and results have been excellent. Patients can immediately see, after their surgery, that the concavity is gone. The final result is evident in about two weeks.

Commonly Asked Questions

How do I determine if my temporal fossa negatively affects my looks? See if your temporal area is too concave. What do we mean by that? Aesthetic impressions come into play in making a judgment, but people who need this procedure generally have more than just a slight depression. The space is severely indented. A proper temporal fossa should be flat or flush

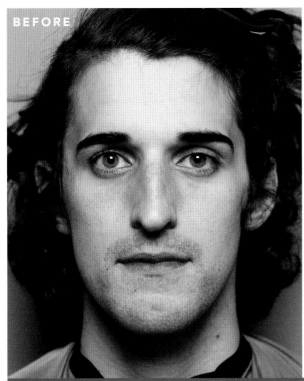

BEFORE

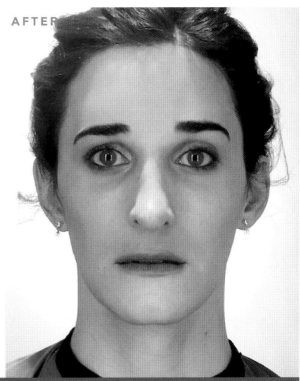

AFTER

This patient underwent fat grafting (injections) to the temples, cheeks, nasolabial folds, and upper and lower lips. Additional procedures include forehead contouring Type III, scalp advancement (hairline lowering), brow lift, rhinoplasty, chin and jawline feminization, and thyroid cartilage reduction (Adam's apple reduction).

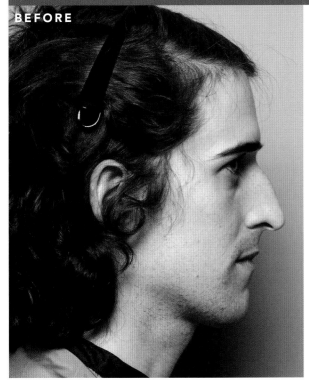

BEFORE

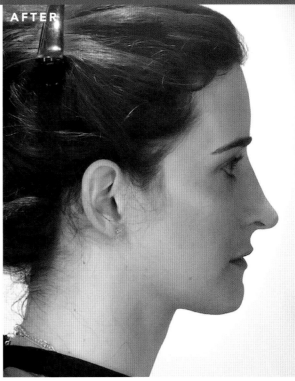

AFTER

with the outside or lateral orbital rims of the eyes. If you are a candidate for this surgery, your depression will be significant, and your face will appear gaunt.

Can methyl methacrylate be injected under the muscle without first elevating it off the underlying bone? We don't think this approach would work. A surgeon would not have control of where the methyl methacrylate might go. Also, correcting any resulting problem could cause significant muscle injury.

Have any of your patients ever been unhappy with the result or even asked you to remove it? No on both counts. Our patients have been extremely happy with the results and have never asked us to remove it.

After the procedure is done, will I need any touch-ups? No. If done correctly, this procedure produces safe, long-lasting, and satisfying results.

Do you prefer methyl methacrylate or fat grafting as the better option for temporal fossa treatment? We tend to prefer fat grafting first in almost all situations. Results are slightly more variable than with methyl methacrylate, but some of the drawbacks of using the resin are avoided. There is less risk for side effects such as infection, for instance. Our results with fat grafting have been very favorable.

A Final Note

Correcting a temporal fossa depression is not necessary for feminizing your face. Many steps can be taken to refine your features without touching the hollows in your temple region. But if your temporal fossa depressions are pronounced rather than shallow, you should consider recontouring them. Supporting the indentations with methyl methacrylate or fat grafting can create more appealing, symmetrical facial contours. These materials offer a safe and permanent solution to a gaunt look.

6

Cheek Contouring

THE SHAPE AND PROMINENCE OF your cheeks, whether they are full or flat, have nothing to do with being female or male. Yet, you may want to consider modifying their contour as part of your facial feminization. Cheeks that are both full and proportioned to your facial features are more aesthetically pleasing than ones that are too narrow or too small. Everyone can benefit from a full cheek profile, but women in particular, look best when their cheeks are full and appropriately prominent.

In this chapter, you will learn how we can enhance your cheekbones with either fat grafting or, less commonly, implants. Whether you are a candidate for reduction or augmentation, contouring your cheeks will definitely enhance your feminized face.

Refining Your Profile

Whatever your gender, reducing or enhancing your cheeks can produce a very positive effect on your overall profile. Yet, not every transfeminine patient needs cheek contouring. Some people are born with a silhouette that no doctor should try to improve. But for other individuals, making changes to this part of the face is both desirable and realistic.

If reshaping the contour will enhance your overall appearance, you and your surgeon should consider it as part of your facial feminization. Whatever you do, your finished cheek profile should not be too full or excessive. Any alteration must be appropriate to your other features. Because a feminine face is smaller than a masculine face, the surrounding areas (the forehead, nose, and mandibular angle) should be feminized (generally reduced in size) before the cheeks are addressed. The cheeks will then become proportionately larger. Whether your surgeon recommends an augmentation or a reduction, the goal should be to keep your face balanced.

Undergoing Cheek Augmentation Surgery

Among transgender individuals, augmenting or enhancing the cheeks is much more common than reducing the cheeks. Surgeons may suggest increasing the fullness to address any small bony cheek prominences left after contouring the surrounding forehead, nose, and mandibular angle. Or they may recommend enhancing

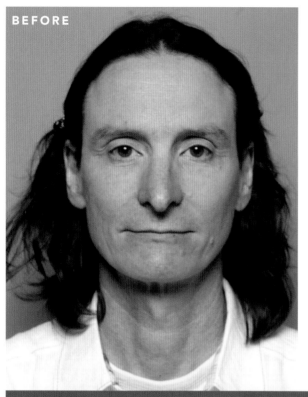

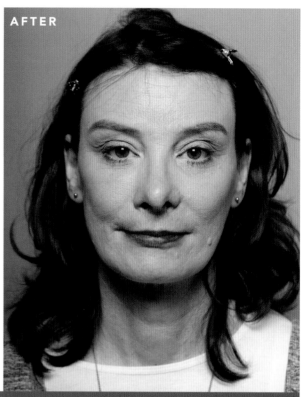

FFS procedures included: Type II forehead contouring, scalp advancement, contouring of the bone surrounding the eyeballs, facial fat grafting, rhinoplasty, upper lip lift, lower jaw contouring with jaw angle reduction, and thyroid cartilage reduction.

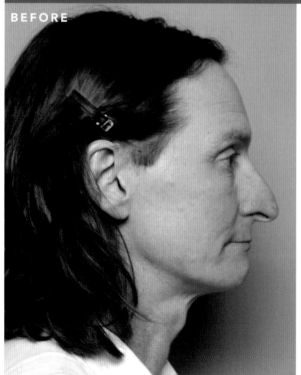

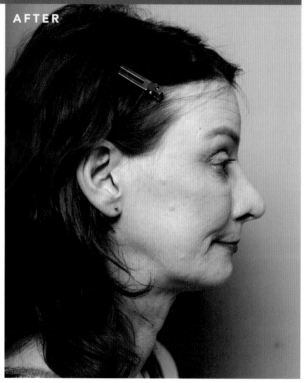

the fullness to rebuild the contours if your cheek fat has dropped with age.

As gravity takes hold, the skin and underlying tissues deflate and then fall, creating the characteristic jowls of an aging face. Many transgender individuals lose significant weight during transition, and older patients tend to lose this weight in the cheeks first. Restoring fullness not only helps correct the contour, but also improves appearance. If you are a younger individual with less than average cheek fat and contour, you can benefit from a similar correction.

Fat Grafting Approach

We have seen a number of patients over the last few years who have been dissatisfied with cheek implants. Patients who need implants often suffer from deflation of the cheeks. It is rare for a cheek implant to be perfectly contoured to the cheeks. Adding a synthetic material that is not perfectly contoured can result in an implant that may be felt or seen through the thin contours of the cheek. In addition, cheek implants do not help with the critical junction between the eyelid and the cheek, which often is a telltale sign of aging. Fat grafting provides your surgeon not only the ability to enhance the cheeks but also to comprehensively restore volume to numerous areas of the face. This volume creates a more balanced appearance that cheek implants alone cannot provide.

Our preferred approach is to use *autologous fat transfer* to enhance the cheeks so that their fullness is a sign of youth and beauty. If the patient feels that they need more augmentation of the skeletal portion of their cheek after a fat transfer procedure, then we will consider placing an implant. Yet, placing an implant where there is inadequate soft tissue coverage is not an ideal approach.

Fat grafting the cheeks is performed under general anesthesia. We perform a very gentle form of liposuction. When we are doing other procedures at the same time, we will do any fat grafting first, because we want the body to be in as natural a state as possible—rather than being swollen from other procedures.

The harvested and processed fat is then loaded into syringes with very small diameter injection cannulas. These *cannulas* are like fine needles, but blunt-tipped devices that allow for placement of fat while reducing the risk of tearing a nerve or blood vessel. Here is where many surgeons fail to use the best technique. The fat must be placed in very small threads or beads so that it can obtain blood supply and vitality from its surrounding tissue to regain circulation. You cannot simply squirt a "blob" of fat into an area of the face and expect it to survive.

During a cheek-contouring procedure, the fat is injected into the cheeks and into the lower eyelids, and blended artistically. This technique preserves and enhances the natural characteristics of your face while augmenting the cheeks. The results are often quite good. We also tend to blend the cheeks and lateral cheek prominences into the temple in combined temporal fossa and cheek augmentations.

Injection of the fat causes the stem cells within it to mobilize. Thus, use of these fat grafts can improve circulation and rejuvenate tissue. We've seen marked improvements in the quality and texture of patients' skin after fat grafting that is apparent by six months after surgery. The quality of the skin continues to improve for one to two years after surgery.

The fat incorporates into the body after it is placed. Usually about 50 to 70 percent of the fat grafts survive; the rate of survival often varies

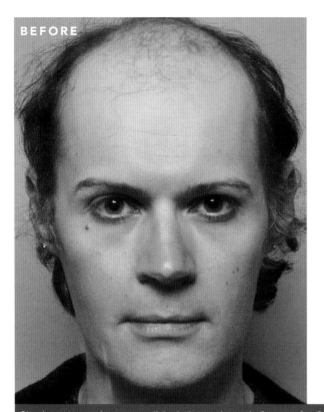

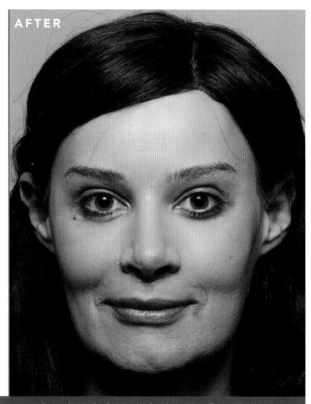

Cheek augmentation accomplished alone using only fat transfer. Other procedures include forehead feminization Type III with rhinoplasty, upper lip lift (vertical shortening), chin and jawline feminization, and thyroid cartilage reduction (Adam's apple reduction).

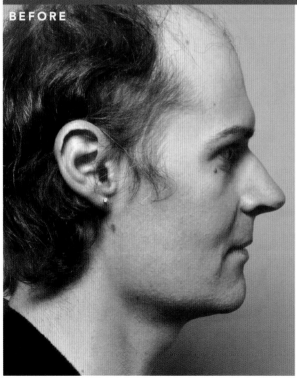

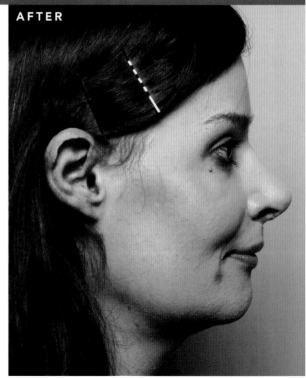

CHEEK IMPLANTS

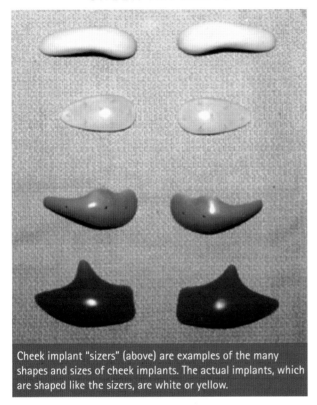

Cheek implant "sizers" (above) are examples of the many shapes and sizes of cheek implants. The actual implants, which are shaped like the sizers, are white or yellow.

from person to person. Although the results can be variable, it is rare for us to have a patient who wishes they had not had their cheeks augmented through fat grafts. The most common complaint we get from our patients is: "I like the augmentation so much that I would like more." In these cases, we can often do more fat grafts later if needed.

Using fat grafts has less risk for side effects than using cheek implants. Rather than introducing a foreign material, we are using the body's own tissue, so there is little inflammatory response. For most cases of cheek augmentation, we use fat grafts as a first-line option because of its many benefits. Occasionally, we will use a cheek implant if one cheek is larger than the other, but that is unusual.

Implant Approach

Cheek augmentations can also be completed with implants, even though bone cuts and repositioning can be useful in some select individuals. Implants are manufactured in many materials, shapes, and thicknesses to accommodate the varied anatomical differences and preferences of individuals.

We usually recommend one of two materials for implants—silicone rubber or high-density polyethylene. Both materials offer durability and compatibility with adjacent tissue. Overall, the results are excellent. After these materials are in place, they stay in place without harming the body.

Silicone Implants. Silicone rubber has been a mainstay material for facial contouring since the mid-1950s. Designed to enhance the soft tissue but not the underlying bone structure, silicone rubber is known for its tissue tolerance. It also is resilient and flexible. Silicone rubber implants are affixed to the bone with tiny screws. We prefer to use screws made of titanium. Although our choice of implants depends on the location and type of cheek deficiency, we often rely on silicone models due to their advantages as implants.

High-Density Polyethylene Implants. Our patients sometimes receive MEDPOR implants, which are made of a lightweight biomaterial, a form of high-density polyethylene, which is a commonly used plastic. The big plus for high-density polyethylene implants is that they rely on tissue integration instead of screws for stability. Occasionally, however, we use a screw for additional reinforcement. A MEDPOR implant can be harder to remove than a silicone model because its porous texture allows for tissue ingrowth. Yet, when positioned correctly, a MEDPOR implant produces excellent long-term

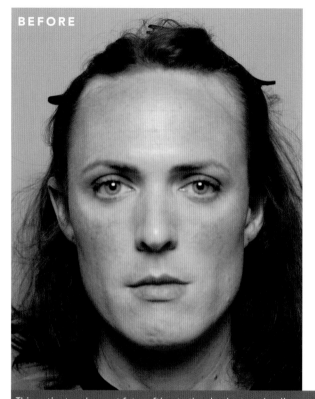

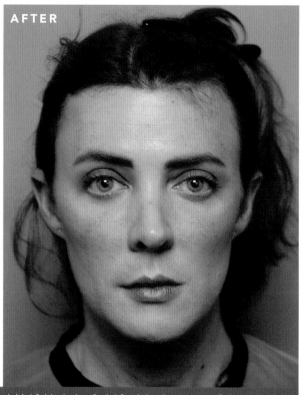

This patient underwent fat grafting to the cheeks, temples, lips, and nasolabial folds during facial feminization surgery. Other procedures include forehead Type III contouring, brow lift, scalp advancement, and rhinoplasty, as well as chin and jawline contouring.

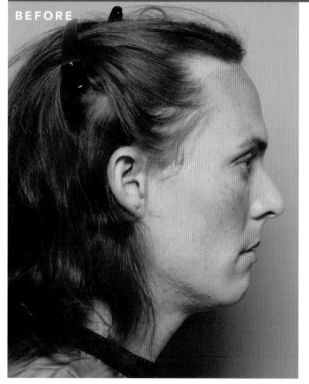

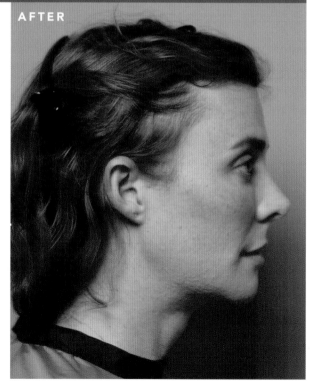

results. For patients who need more fullness in the lower cheek, MEDPOR works well.

Custom Option. In recent times, it has become possible to build custom-made implants that are tailored to your individual anatomy. A CT scan is required and from that scan a model is made of the skull and an implant can be fabricated. These are usually good options for asymmetrical issues where one side does not match the other. This method is quite costly, and these implants cost four times what an "off-the-shelf" implant might cost. Our opinion is that these options are occasionally very useful, but should be limited to special or unusual cases.

Other Implant Options. Your surgeon may offer other options. Medical implants today come in many different materials. Some doctors use *hydroxyapatite*, a synthetic bone made from altered coral. Some doctors advise injecting hyaluronic acid, collagen, and other materials. However, we are not a fan of these approaches, because fillers must be repeated over the years. To be clear, they are effective options for short-term results. The long-term cost, however, may be higher because of the need for repeat injections. However, these types of options can be especially useful for patients who do not want to undergo surgery.

Cheek Implant Procedure

Cheek augmentations can be performed under either general or local anesthesia on an outpatient basis. If other procedures are being completed at the same time, however, they'll likely be done under general anesthesia.

To place a *malar*, or cheekbone implant, we make an incision through the *buccal mucosa*, the mucous membrane inside the cheek. We then lift the soft tissue directly over the malar prominence,

the most prominent part of the cheekbone, to create a pocket. The implant is slipped in and then stabilized using one or two titanium screws.

After the minute fibers of a MEDPOR model grab the tissue, the implant is positioned permanently. Silicone implants, however, are almost always held in place with tiny screws.

The success rate for cosmetic improvement with cheek augmentation is virtually 100 percent. Our patients are routinely happy with their outcomes. On rare occasions, some patients may want a change in thickness or shape.

We are usually happy to provide the desired fullness, but not if it gives the face an extreme look. As with any other cosmetic procedure, a cheek implant should be proportional to the rest of your face.

When Not to Augment the Cheeks

Cheek augmentation should not be performed if adjacent areas of the face have not been properly reduced in size during feminization. Clearly, female faces are smaller than male faces, so if you plan to undergo transition, your surgeon must properly decrease your forehead, nose, and lower jaw first. Then, you and your surgeon can address cheek augmentation.

If your forehead, nose, and jaw are not properly reshaped, your cheeks may continue to look too small. Some surgeons routinely use augmentation to compensate for both this imbalance and their inability to properly feminize the surrounding features. For instance, instead of adequately taking down the forehead and reducing the nose, some surgeons build up the cheeks to make the face look more proportional. Such a maneuver only increases the facial size rather than reducing it and normally does not produce an aesthetically pleasing result.

Undergoing Cheek Reduction Surgery

Cheek reduction is not a common procedure in transgender Caucasian, Hispanic, or African American individuals. It is not unusual, however, in Asians, particularly Korean and Chinese patients, whose wide cheek structures are part of their ethnicity. In some of these individuals, a broader facial look is regarded as very attractive; in others, it is considered the opposite. The few transgender patients and other individuals we have treated with cheek reduction have been Asians who want the fullness without the wide facial appearance.

Fortunately, we can accommodate these individuals with either of two techniques. The first involves using a special drill to burr down or shave the excess bone at the *zygomatic arch*, the bony ridge that extends from beneath the eye socket sideways to the temples. The second requires cutting out an appropriate amount of the zygomatic anterior arch, rotating or turning the malar cheek inward, and securing it with a small plate and two tiny screws. Neither the plate nor the screws can be felt outside the skin. Both approaches may be necessary in some individuals, depending on the problem. Your surgeon will consider the shape and thickness of the bony arch and the extent of its lateral protrusion in making the decision. After a smaller contour is achieved, the incisions are closed with sutures.

After Your Augmentation or Reduction Surgery

The recovery after cheek augmentation or reduction surgery is quick and usually uneventful. If these procedures are performed with other facial feminization techniques, there will be some postoperative care overlap. You still should pay close attention to the following specifics about recovery and possible complications. This information will help make cheek-contouring surgery a success.

Recovery and Follow-up Care

The sutures your surgeon places in the mouth will dissolve. There are no dressings for this part of your feminization surgery, so showering will not be an issue, unless you are undergoing additional procedures that require external bandages. Taking the entire course of your prescription antibiotic is extremely important in keeping any infections at bay. But also pay attention to the following.

Diet

You will need to stay on a soft food diet for at least ten to twelve days to protect your incision. We tell our patients to avoid meat, sandwiches, and fruits (such as apples) or vegetables (such as carrots) that are tough to bite into and chew. Instead, we recommend soups, mashed potatoes, and easy-to-swallow choices.

Oral Care

During recovery, you must brush your teeth at least three times a day to remove bacteria from your mouth. When you brush, you will probably experience some tenderness around the incision lines in your gums. So, take it easy.

Activity

The guidelines for physical activity after cheek surgery are the same as for other facial feminization procedures: Refrain from physical activity for ten to fourteen days and then build up your routine slowly. If your face is swollen after minimal exercise, hold off a little longer. If you work at home, you can return to your job the next day. Otherwise, you should wait up to ten to twelve days. Keep your fingers off your face and avoid touching your cheeks to see how they feel.

Sleeping Habits

After any facial procedure, you cannot lie flat on your back immediately. Cheek surgery is no different. You will need to sleep with your head elevated to prevent the swelling from getting worse. For a period of three to four weeks, patients who undergo whole face feminizations usually support their heads during sleep. If your surgery involves only an implant, you can reduce this time to fourteen days. Our patients often sleep on wedges or on three to four pillows.

Side Effects and Potential Complications

Pain, bruising, and swelling are not big issues with cheek surgery. Expect some discomfort, and you may need pain medication for a few days. Although your lower eyelid may turn black and blue, the discoloration is usually not significant. There is one caveat with augmentation: Some porous implants, such as MEDPOR, can irritate the tissues and cause more temporary swelling than silicone implants. Even then, however, swelling will diminish or disappear in several weeks. It should not interfere with your daily life.

Fat grafts are even less likely to cause side effects than implants. Infections are unlikely because the cheeks are being augmented with your own tissue. As mentioned previously, this makes it unlikely that the body will mount an inflammatory response to the grafts. What other issues can cause problems after cheek surgery? The following are several you need to consider.

Asymmetry

No matter what facial surgery you undergo, your surgeon may have to improve any preexisting asymmetry, or a lack of balance from one side to the other. Most of us are asymmetrical or uneven to some degree. One cheek is not the perfect mirror image of the other. Your surgeon, however, will, and should make every effort to ensure that your cheeks show improved symmetry or look relatively the same after the procedure. Human beings rarely have perfect symmetry, and perfect symmetry of facial features is usually perceived as a disturbing feature for most people. Beyond a certain threshold, lack of symmetry, or asymmetry, also begins to be so unusual as to become a problem. Fortunately, in most cases, we can produce a beautiful and appropriately symmetric appearance.

Infections

Infections are rare with cheek implants, but they can occur. Because your surgeon is introducing foreign material into your body through the mouth, you will be prescribed an antibiotic to prevent any problems. If, however, an infection develops despite this medication, the implants may have to be removed. Fortunately, the body tolerates oral bacteria extremely well. Every time you brush your teeth, for instance, microbes enter your bloodstream through your mouth, and are dealt with very effectively. Not so with skin bacteria; they are not tolerated as well by the body.

Because it is easier to contract an infection through your skin during or after a facial procedure, stop any electrolysis treatment to remove hair four weeks prior to surgery to three months afterward. Even though sterile needles are used in the process, bacteria around the hair follicles can enter the bloodstream and infect any recent surgical site. Remove that risk by temporarily avoiding electrolysis, waxing, or plucking hair anywhere on your body for three months.

Numbness

Temporary numbness can occur with cheek augmentation or reduction. After implant surgery, some patients report numbness on the side of the nose, in the upper lip, and over the cheek. It occurs because the *infraorbital nerve,* the prominent sensory nerve in the region, is stretched or otherwise injured during the procedure. Normal sensation returns in a few weeks. Patients may also complain of difficulty speaking or smiling, as well as funny sensations when they yawn or chew. Much of that is due to stiffness from swelling in the cheeks. These sensations pass within days. Some numbness to the lateral side of the cheek can occur because the surgeon usually cuts the *zygomaticofacial nerve,* a sensory nerve in the middle of the cheek. Patients rarely experience this numbness, however, most likely because the surrounding nerves compensate for any loss of feeling.

A partial, temporary, or permanent upper facial paralysis might occur if your surgeon cuts or otherwise injures the temporal branch of the seventh nerve as it crosses the zygomatic arch. This nerve helps lift your brow when you express surprise or lowers it when you express confusion. This damage can possibly be repaired by reconnecting the nerve endings, although the surgery is very involved. Using Botox on the other side of the face may also help. Fortunately, paralysis is very rare. We have seen paralysis in only one patient who underwent cheek reduction.

Outcome of Surgery

Most patients are pleased with the outcome of their cheek surgery. Cheek augmentation and reduction usually yields a satisfying result for patients. Still, be sure to discuss with your surgeon the look you want to achieve by augmenting or reducing your cheeks before the procedure. Be prepared to describe or even show pictures of the outcome you'd like. By identifying the best options for your facial structure, your surgeon will be able to give you an appropriate cheekbone contour that meets your expectations. Hopefully, with the right choices, you will need this surgery only once.

Commonly Asked Questions

Do you use soft tissue injectable fillers to augment the cheeks? We like them in cases where surgery is not being performed, or if a small touch-up is needed after surgery. We think that in the long run, using filler materials is not cost-effective for most patients, because a large amount may be necessary, and repeated treatments can be expensive. However, many who are not quite ready for surgery find this a great option.

What happens if the implant gets infected and must be removed? What will the cheeks look like? Rarely, cheek implants must be removed due to infection. When that happens, the cheeks may sag a little, because they are no longer supported from underneath. Initially, we create a pocket for each implant by lifting the soft tissue off the underlying bone. After the implant is removed, however, the capsule that normally forms around it does not immediately reattach to the bone. (It may never do so.) Without that underlying support, the cheeks can drop. Fixing the sagging may require a new implant, fat graft, or cheek lift, in which the cheek tissues are elevated and tightened.

Are there any special conditions that make cheek implantation difficult and fat transfer more desirable? Yes, being HIV positive can be problematic. The condition itself is not an issue. About twenty-five or thirty of our transgender patients are HIV positive. Although protease inhibitors, the antiviral medications patients take to treat HIV, are very effective, they can cause cheek fat loss. They may also reduce the number and function of blood platelets—circulating cell fragments necessary for normal clotting.

To compensate for their hollow mid-face appearance, patients on protease inhibitors often desire cheek augmentation. Although the procedure is usually successful, the platelet issues connected to the drugs put these patients at risk for blood pooling *(hematoma)* around a cheek implant. If this area then gets infected, which can occur in these cases, the implant may need to be removed.

This example is one of several reasons why we have a strong preference for fat transfer. There is less risk for infection and hematomas, even in patients on protease inhibitors. Because the problem in these cases is fat loss, the solution should be fat addition—rather than adding implants. Replace like with like, is a time-tested plastic surgery adage.

If you are on protease inhibitors, make sure to address any concerns and your options with your surgeon. Fortunately, the use of protease inhibitors does not seem to be an issue for other facial feminization procedures.

A Final Note

There is no such thing as a "masculine" or "feminine" cheek. Whatever your gender, your face looks better when your cheeks are full, and also proportional to your other features. Compared to cheek augmentation, cheek reduction is rare among transgender individuals, but, when needed, it can improve your overall profile. Cheek augmentation is not a facial feminization procedure, but one that can enhance your overall look.

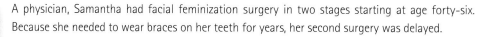

A physician, Samantha had facial feminization surgery in two stages starting at age forty-six. Because she needed to wear braces on her teeth for years, her second surgery was delayed.

WHAT PROCEDURES DID YOU HAVE DONE?

The first stage was scalp advancement, forehead, eyebrow lift, nose job, lip lift, and thyroid cartilage reduction. Because I had *micrognathia* (small jaw), my chin used to sit way back and I had a very bad overbite. Prior to my second stage, my teeth needed braces for almost three years so they would line up after my *BSSO,* or *bilateral sagittal split osteotomy.* Dr. Deschamps-Braly cut my lower jaw sagittally, just behind the teeth, in order to slide the jaw forward.

HOW DID YOU DECIDE ON YOUR SURGEON?

Because I'm a physician, and because there were other things that needed to be done for work simultaneously, I did a lot of planning ahead. My hospital did not want me to practice under one name and present differently, so I timed all my identity documents to change during my FFS medical leave.

I treated my research like a medical school project. I looked into all trans medical procedures to prioritize which would be important to me first. Because I see patients every day, I felt that my face was the most important thing for me to do first.

I did research on quite a few doctors for several months, looking at sites where people could upload their photos. Some other surgeons post results on their sites. Given my medical background, I was able to look up malpractice claims, number of cases, who trained the surgeons, education, and board certifications. I narrowed it down very quickly.

Dr. Ousterhout is a founder of FFS, so his knowledge transfer to Dr. Deschamps-Braly speaks volumes. Dr. Deschamps-Braly and I are both very analytical, but with an appreciation for art, flow, design, and aesthetics. At the same time, we both have a profound appreciation for precision and attention to detail. We went over my radiographs, and he made some drawings and showed some computer-generated mock-ups. After my consultation, I had a really good feeling, so I went with them.

My only in-person consultation was in 2016, with both Dr. Ousterhout and Dr. Deschamps-Braly. I completely deferred to them on what would be best for my face. I knew that I wanted my face to look more feminine, and that was really about it. I didn't connect with the person I saw in the mirror, and I always felt as if I'd been living in someone else's body. I wanted them to bring out the person underneath. It's like the quote often attributed to Michelangelo about sculpting the statue of David: Just chip away the stone that doesn't look like David. I was always there, and Dr. Deschamps-Braly simply chipped away the bones and other things that weren't me. I consider him my Michelangelo!

WHAT WAS RECOVERY LIKE?

I had a headache the first night, and the first few days were a blur, but it was not as bad as I expected. Getting the nose stent removed after a week was uncomfortable, and my swelling peaked around that time. Even with the swelling, when I looked in the mirror, I was overwhelmed. I cried out of joy because I didn't see the other person any more.

I didn't have a lot of pain. I didn't have any issues. Perhaps doing it in two stages made recovery easier than those who can do everything at once. When I returned to work after five weeks, I still had some swelling, but I was presentable. In fact, I looked younger because I didn't have any wrinkles! I had some residual swelling for several months.

The numbness was not a problem, but it lasted longer than I had expected. I had some numbness in my right lower lip and chin for about six months before it came back to normal. The second surgery left the masseter muscles very tight, and I had to do a few weeks of uncomfortable exercises to be able to unclench my jaw and open my mouth wide again.

Because he couldn't do it until the BSSO healed, Dr. Deschamps-Braly would like to do a third stage where he smooths the jawbone where the BSSO cut was made. But that's because he's a perfectionist. It's not something I am too concerned about. He can do it when he does my facelift!

WHAT ADVICE DO YOU HAVE FOR OTHERS CONSIDERING FACIAL FEMINIZATION?

First and foremost, do your research. Everyone is different. Your genetics, family traits, and underlying conditions will all affect how you recover from your surgery. Not only should your doctor be competent, but you should also have a good rapport. That will help with your recovery and so forth.

Your results may not be quite the same as everyone else's. Don't think, "Well, so-and-so had a really good result, and that's how I want my face to look." Your bone structure is different than that person, so your outcome is going to be different. Sometimes, people set themselves up with the wrong expectations, then they perceive that they had a "bad" outcome when in fact they had a really good outcome. It may not be what they expected, but it's the outcome their body was able to produce. Having your expectations well aligned with reality is a good thing.

HOW HAS FACIAL FEMINIZATION CHANGED YOUR LIFE?

I don't know if there are really words for that. Because I was bullied as a child about my chin, I was very self-conscious about it my whole life. So even though it wasn't specifically about gender, the chin work was what had the most profound impact for me. The confidence to be myself and smile and be happy are great, but the bonus of not having that chin and being reminded of that grade school bullying has been the blessing of my lifetime.

The most pleasant surprise is how often I get complimented on my nose. A lot of people think I have a cute nose now, and I wasn't expecting that. A lot of people compliment me on my smile, which is also thanks to my orthodontist. Before transition, when anyone would give me a compliment, I couldn't just take the compliment. I would always make an excuse about why I didn't look good. The root of that was because I didn't like myself. I'm now learning to take compliments, which is nice. Now when someone compliments me, I just smile and say, "Thank you!"

I feel blessed for the life I've had. I just wish more of it would have been as this me. My professional interactions are largely unchanged. I'm still the same with friends, even though many are new friends. The big change is that I smile a lot more because I'm happier. I'm more compassionate. I'm more loving. I'm more giving. I'm like a flower that has bloomed. That's what facial feminization and being myself did for me.

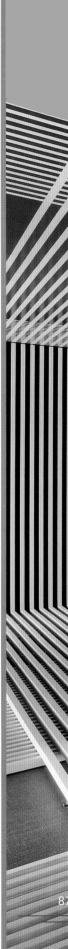

7

Nose Reshaping

NOTHING DEFINES YOUR APPEARANCE quite like your nose. Like it or not, people identify you, and even judge you, by its shape and size. If your nose overwhelms your other features, it can hamper your self-confidence. That's especially true if you are transitioning from male to female. Having a nose that is bigger and wider than the smaller, narrowed version found in most women can affect the feminine identity you wish to project. Can it be changed? Yes. Reshaping your nose plays an important part in facial feminization.

Differences in Male and Female Noses

If you're a transgender individual, your nose can challenge your femininity. Distinct differences are found between the sexes. Masculine noses are usually larger than feminine noses. The male nose is often longer and wider with larger nostrils and bulkier tips than the female nose. A masculine nose either points ahead or slightly downward, while a feminine nose will often point slightly upward. Having a slightly upturned nose, in fact, is considered a mark of femininity. In some ethnicities, the bridge of the female nose—or the bony ridge at the top of the nose—may scoop or dip before sloping downward or into a slightly upturned tip.

Men also have sharper angles between the nose and forehead and between the nose and upper lip. The profile of the cartoon character Dick Tracy is an example. You may not have his chiseled profile, but your nose probably projects off your forehead more abruptly than most women's noses. You may even have an unsightly bump, called a *dorsal hump,* on your nose.

In changing your nose to fit your new gender, your surgeon's goal is to make sure that it slopes gently from your forehead and is free of bumps. He or she will also reduce the size of your nose and sculpt it, so that it fully reflects your new identity. Reshaping the nose may also add to your beauty as well as your femininity.

Ethnic Differences

Noses are a product of ethnic and genetic makeup, but can also be affected by injury, trauma, or birth defects. Your surgeon will have to keep all these individual differences in mind when performing a rhinoplasty.

Women of northern European descent frequently have a straight or slightly concave, or scooped, nasal bridge. Females of Middle Eastern descent, however, tend to have nasal bridges that are more convex or bulge forward. African American nasal structures are wider than those of Caucasians, and their bridges are flatter. Asian noses don't have a significant bridge, and their nostrils don't flare out much.

In our experience, the goal of facial feminization—including changes to the nose—is not to adhere to a Caucasian standard of beauty. Women of color, including our transgender patients, usually opt for a scaled-down version of their existing noses. Building up the bridge is a common request, too. Whatever we do, we make sure the nose fits with other facial features and reflects the patient's desires.

Skin Type

The changes made to your nose in rhinoplasty may sometimes be limited by the thickness of your skin. If you have thin skin, your surgeon can significantly reduce the size of your nose, because the skin can be draped easily over the reshaped framework underneath. But if your skin is thick, your doctor may not be able to do nearly as much remodeling as you might like. Because thick skin is more difficult to control, it doesn't adapt easily to new contours. Although your doctor will be able to improve your nasal structure markedly, your new nose may not be as small as you envision.

Also, be aware that your doctor cannot narrow the nasal passages too much, because the underlying framework must be preserved to permit normal breathing. Even so, your basic nasal appearance after a rhinoplasty will be more feminine than it once was.

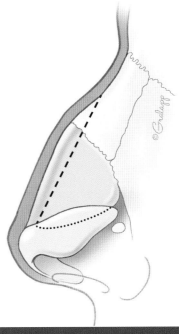

Example of a common nose profile and the surgical approach to reshaping the nose. The dotted lines show areas where bone and cartilage will be removed.

Selecting a Nose that Fits Your Face

Should you choose your new nose from a photograph? We encourage patients to bring us photos of noses they admire when we consult with them about their surgeries. It's helpful to have both side and frontal views because you'll want to see what you may look like from the front and in profile. Yet, it is unethical for us or any other surgeon to promise that rhinoplasty can replicate the image precisely. When you bring us some good photos, we can discuss them and what is realistic for your surgery.

Most importantly, we think that it is crucial for a patient to annotate, or make notes about, the photos of noses that you show to us. This helps us to understand your thinking. Before we asked patients for this, we would often receive pictures of vastly different noses from a patient saying: "I want something like this." When we'd

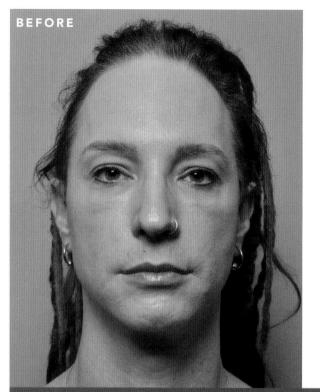

BEFORE

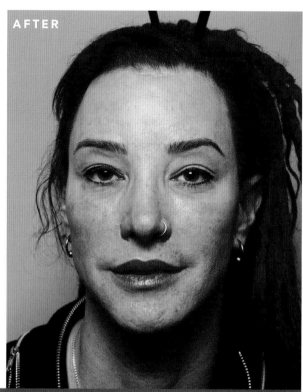

AFTER

Patient had a feminizing rhinoplasty in addition to the following procedures: scalp advancement (hairline lowering), forehead Type III feminization, pan facial fat grafting, chin feminization, open rhino/septoplasty, and upper lip lift with augmentation using fat injections.

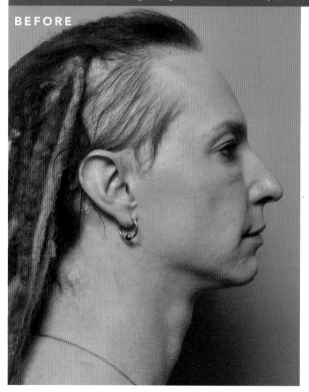

BEFORE

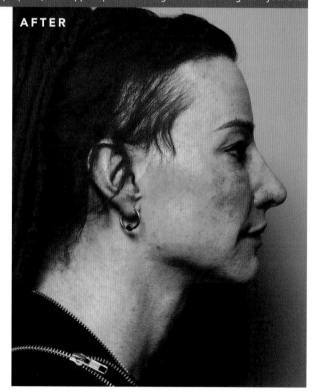

AFTER

point out that the noses are vastly different, the patient often concedes that they just thought the person's nose was pretty. Annotating the photos makes you think about the features of a nose that you want to have.

As surgeons, we cannot turn a big nose with thick skin into a perky profile. On the other hand, someone with thin skin may be well positioned to achieve that very look. The point is that plastic surgeons must work with what's already there. So yes, bring photos of your ideal nose, but be open to a different profile.

Undergoing Nasal Feminization Surgery

Rhinoplasty is one of the most common of all plastic surgery procedures. Derived from the Greek term, "rhino," meaning nose, and "plasty," meaning to form or shape, this procedure allows surgeons to alter the look and correct any mechanical or structural problem involving the nose. To perform the surgery, your doctor will remove, shift, and/or modify the underlying structural bone and cartilage.

Your surgeon can reduce the size, narrow the width, straighten the bridge, reshape the tip, shorten the nostrils, and remove any bumps. Your surgeon can also revise any angles or curves that impact the nose's relationship with other parts of the face. Surgeons can straighten a crooked nasal septum, the bone and cartilage partition between your right and left nasal cavities. And if they are obstructive, your *turbinates,* the wing-like airway structures that help moisten the air you breathe, can also be reduced or repositioned.

You may not need every improvement we've mentioned to achieve a more feminine contour. Yet, because a refined nasal profile is important to most women, you may want to

undergo a nasal feminization. Rhinoplasty is perhaps the most individualized operation in plastic surgery, which means it's also one of the most difficult to perform. Surgeons must accommodate the unique angles, bends, and curves of a patient's nasal anatomy. At the same time, they must navigate through the nose's complicated structural parts—skin, bones, cartilage, mucous membranes, blood vessels, and nerves—to preserve nasal function.

Whatever your gender, each surgery presents its own set of challenges, and each outcome yields its own rewards. By tailoring your nose with established techniques, your surgeon can not only protect your nasal function, but also create a smaller, distinctively feminine structure.

Addressing the Nose and Forehead Together

We often insist that nasal surgery should be performed along with forehead feminization, if you need both. As you reconcile your facial features with your new gender, the relationship between your forehead and nose becomes increasingly important. You want them to be proportional to each other and to reflect the gentle angles of a female profile. Performing these surgeries together also reduces the risk of potential problems after surgery.

When performing these procedures together, your surgeon will probably set your forehead back (often by just several millimeters) behind your nose at the *radix,* the bony triangular junction where the forehead and nose meet. This usually can't be achieved with a rhinoplasty alone.

We discussed forehead contouring in greater detail in chapter 4, but by doing it in tandem with a rhinoplasty, we can ensure an appropriate transition between the nose and forehead. After repositioning the lower forehead, we then shave down the bony radix and preserve its union with the nose. To ensure a clearer view during this maneuver, we prefer an *open rhinoplasty*. In an open rhinoplasty, the surgeon approaches the nose from the outside, making a small incision in the *columella,* or the fleshy external end of the bridge that divides the nose. As a result, we can set back the forehead-to-nose juncture effectively and safely.

Some surgeons may try to convince you that they can do the nose first and the forehead later, or vice versa, but that is not recommended.

Inpatient Procedure

Nasal surgery is often completed as an outpatient procedure. Yet, nasal feminization, particularly when combined with forehead feminization, needs to be performed as an inpatient operation under general anesthesia. This usually

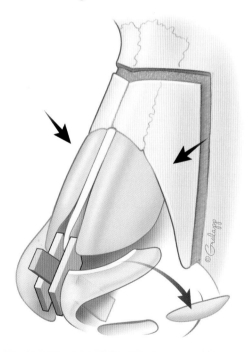

Illustration depicting the various surgical modifications to the nose during rhino/septoplasty to narrow the nose. A strip may be removed from the cartilage that runs down the center of the nose and cartilage may be trimmed from both sides.

requires one night in the hospital. We personally would not conceive of doing a rhinoplasty under local anesthesia, given the complexity of the procedure and the fact that there is a certain amount of bleeding. We want our patients to be completely comfortable and breathing normally during the process. Using general anesthesia is now the safest and most effective way to put a patient under during surgery on the nose.

Open vs. Closed Rhinoplasties

Nose surgeries are performed with either a *closed rhinoplasty,* an endonasal approach, in which the surgeon performs the entire procedure within the nose, or an *open rhinoplasty* (or external approach). Both techniques rely on strategically placed incisions to gain access to the underlying bone and cartilage. The approach depends on both the complexity of your case and your surgeon's preferences. We like the open approach, but first let's quickly review the more traditional closed procedure. Until the 1990s, it was the routine technique for most nose reshaping surgeries.

Closed Rhinoplasty. The biggest plus of a closed rhinoplasty is that it does not leave an external scar on the columella. Instead, the surgeon works entirely inside the nose, making incisions within the nostrils and nasal cavities. In skilled hands, this technique can yield many reshaping possibilities. But there are drawbacks.

In a closed rhinoplasty, the surgeon has a limited view and ability to manipulate the bone and cartilage. This means that the closed approach may not be the best choice for complicated initial procedures or revision surgeries. We use this approach in about 2 percent of all rhinoplasties.

Open Rhinoplasty. The major benefit of an "open" technique is the visibility a surgeon

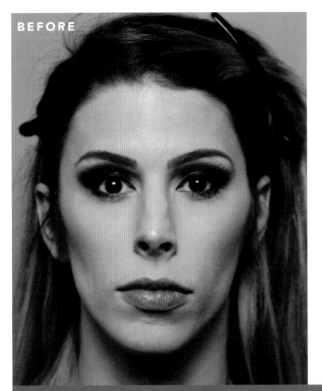

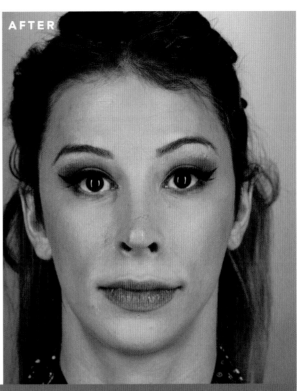

This patient underwent a feminizing rhinoplasty with a 6 mm reduction to the bridge of her nose to reduce the height and width. Other procedures include forehead feminization with forehead Type III contouring, brow lift, chin and jawline feminization, and thyroid cartilage reduction (Adam's apple reduction).

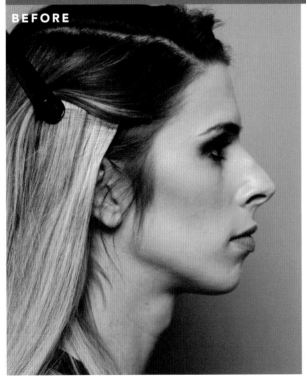

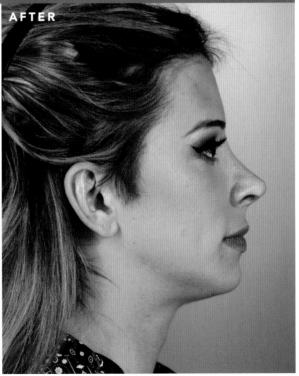

SURGICAL STEPS FOR NARROWING THE TIP OF THE NOSE

WIDE TIP

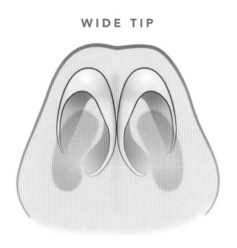

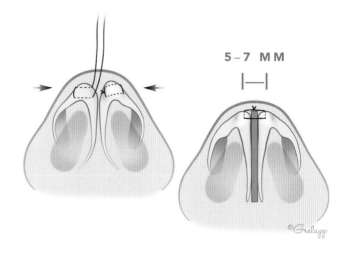

5-7 MM

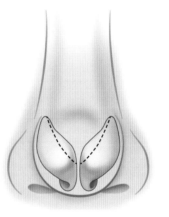

All five images show techniques used to narrow an excessively wide tip of the nose. The two lower images include removing cartilage in addition to suture techniques in order to narrow the tip.

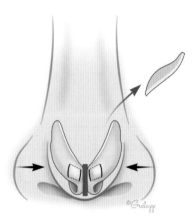

has of the entire nose. With this approach, the surgeon makes an initial incision across the columella (the bridge of cartilage and bone that divides the nostrils). Although there are several ways to open the *columella*, the surgeon chooses which cut will produce the best scar. Subsequent incisions are made inside the nasal cavity to allow the surgeon to lift the skin and expose the bone and cartilage. This maneuver provides a clear view of the underlying structures, much like lifting the hood of a car to see the engine.

We use this technique in 98 percent of our rhinoplasties. It gives us the flexibility to sculpt a very pleasing profile that we can refine precisely along the way. With an open technique, it's easier to control bleeding, position the bony supports of the nose, correct septal deformities, reduce tip fullness and asymmetries, and insert cartilage grafts. Of course, there are downsides to the open approach. You may have increased swelling in addition to a small scar on the outside of your columella. But the puffiness will diminish with healing, and the scar will fade over time. This technique is the best option for most rhinoplasties, especially challenging surgeries on transfeminine patients.

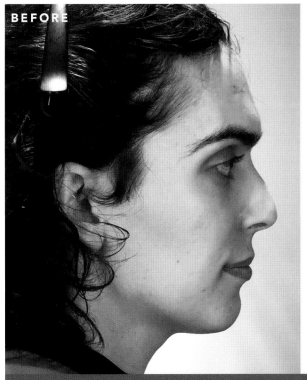

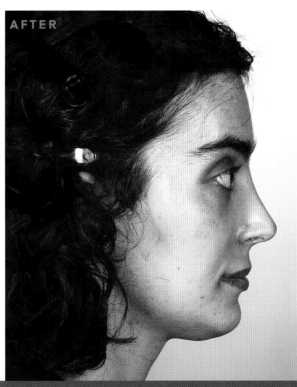

An open rhinoplasty and septoplasty surgery corrected this patient's dorsal hump and downward pointed tip. The patient simultaneously underwent forehead contouring (type III) , scalp advancement (hairline lowering) , brow lift, and chin feminization.

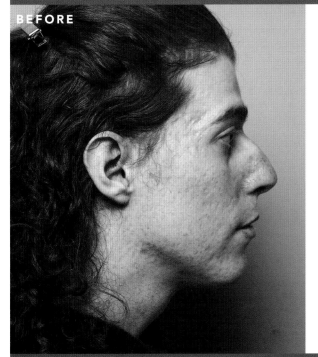

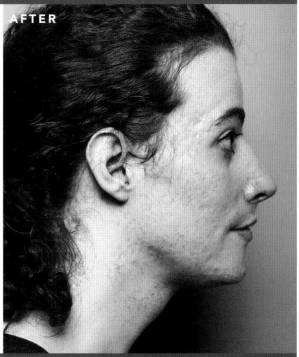

This patient underwent rhinoplasty and septoplasty to correct bone and cartilage structures between the nostrils. Other FFS procedures: scalp elevation, upper lip lift, chin and jaw feminization, thyroid cartilage reduction and, facial fat grafting.

REDUCING THE ALAR

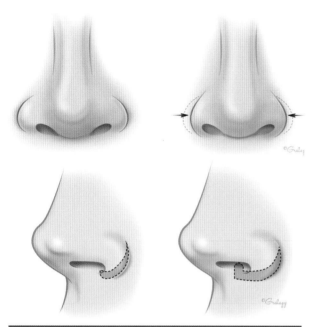

Placement of surgical incisions made to reduce the outside rims of the nostrils. The procedure narrows the width of the lower portion of the nose.

Other Factors Your Surgeon Will Consider

After the underlying framework of nasal bones, septum, and cartilage is exposed by either approach, the surgeon must ensure that your finished nose is straight, symmetrical, and complements your other feminine facial features. In doing so the surgeon concentrates on four major areas:

- *Nasal dorsum and dorsal hump.* Your surgeon will resize and reshape the nasal dorsum, the ridge that runs vertically from the top of your nose to the tip. Your surgeon will also remove any cartilage or bone that forms a dorsal hump, a major detraction on many male faces. Because most women don't have this noticeable bump midway between the tip and bridge, it should be eliminated. The nasal bones must also be cut at their base and narrowed.

- *Nasal septum and turbinates.* Your surgeon will remove any deformed portions of the bone and cartilage (the septum) separating the right and left air passages. The surgeon may also reduce any enlarged *turbinates*, the narrow, long curved bones that divide the airway into four passages. An enlarged and/or deformed septum and turbinates can block your airways, so repairing them will help you breathe and sleep easier.

- *Tip of the nose.* To feminize the tip of the nose, your surgeon may reduce the size, improve the shape, shorten the length or projection, or change the angle. By removing and/or refining the excess cartilage that makes a male nose tip wider or larger, your surgeon can create the smaller, slightly upwardly tip of a feminine nose. Your surgeon will also ensure that the tip is proportional to the rest of your face.

- *Nostrils.* Nostrils tend to be smaller in women than in men, so reducing the *alar* or outside rims to decrease the flare will no doubt be part of your feminization surgery. Surgeons have several ways to narrow the nostril so that the scars heal inconspicuously over time. The result is a more tailored, pleasing feminine look.

After completing these steps, incisions are stitched closed with sutures that dissolve in about a week. The dressing that will most likely be used on your nose is made up of a plaster cast, a splint, and tape. Along with a chin dressing, the nose dressing must be kept dry. You also want to avoid any bumps on the nose or other accidents. The cast is removed in six to eight days. We also tape a small gauze piece beneath the nostrils to collect any nasal mucous drips. After surgery, you'll breathe mostly through your mouth for at least five days. Although you may be a little uncomfortable, the results will be worth it.

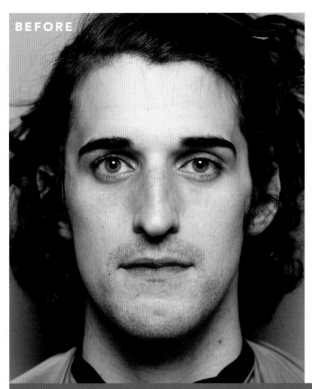

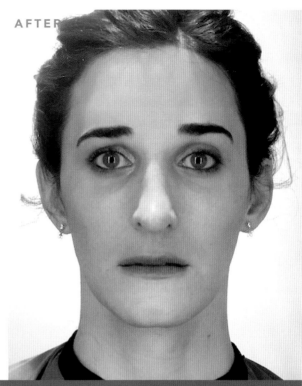

On the left, before rhinoplasty and septoplasty to reshape bone and cartilage structures between the nostrils. On the right, notice the reduction in both the size and shape of the nose; the nose also has a slight upturn. Other FFS procedures: Type III forehead contouring, scalp advancement, brow lift, chin and jaw feminization, thyroid cartilage reduction, and facial fat grafting.

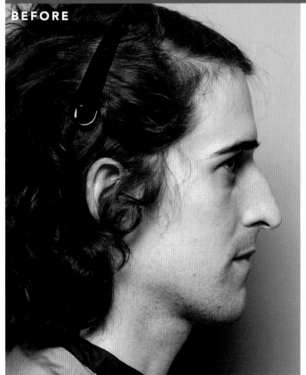

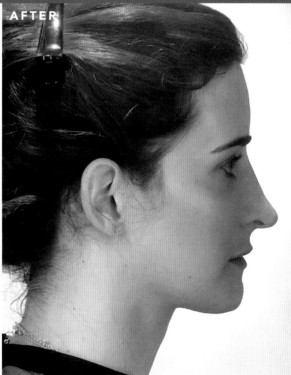

Secondary Surgery

Due to its complexity, rhinoplasty is associated with a high percentage of unfavorable results, such as a small scar, bony prominence, or slight asymmetry. Usually, these problems can be corrected with a minor surgical repair. Follow-up surgical repair is necessary if the:

- *bony radix*—the bridge of the nose—remains too full after the first surgery to be aesthetically pleasing

- *columella*—the bridge of cartilage and bone that divides the nostrils—is hanging too far below the alar rims of the nostrils after the first surgery

- *nasal supra tip*—the area about 10 mm above the actual tip—is too full after the first surgery

- *nasal tip*—is still too bulky or wide after the initial surgery

- *alar rims*—the outside borders of the nostrils—are too wide after the initial surgery

- *nose looks too asymmetrical*

We can usually correct an asymmetrical nose during a second operation. Yet, if the problem existed before the first procedure, and we corrected it once, there is a fair chance that it will return. Why? When the nose is off to one side for a long time, there's less skin on that side. Because the skin has memory, it continually works to pull the nose back to its original position. Eventually it succeeds.

Twenty-three percent of our FFS rhinoplasty patients have had a previous procedure completed elsewhere, but most of their noses are still too masculine. Prior to our follow-up surgery, the noses of these patients were usually still too large and were not appropriately proportional for their new feminine forehead. Some of their surgeons were not told that the patient was changing gender, so placing a little

nose adjacent to a large masculine forehead would have looked inappropriate. A revision or initial rhinoplasty is crucial for most patients who seek a forehead feminization.

It's important to keep in mind that a certain number of every plastic surgeon's nose patients return for revisions. The published rhinoplasty revision rate among our colleagues is between 8 and 19 percent. We currently have a revision rate of less than 4 percent. The more important and reassuring news for our transfeminine patients is that these issues, if they occur, can usually be corrected with a second procedure.

After Your Nasal Feminization Surgery

Our nasal feminization patients begin their recovery with one night in the hospital following surgery if they are also undergoing other gender confirmation procedures of the face. We do not routinely keep rhinoplasty-only patients in the hospital overnight. We see them after surgery and the next morning.

We have a different philosophy than many of our colleagues who put the smallest bandage on the nose. We place a large dressing on nose surgery patients because we want them to remember that they've had surgery and that they need to be careful during their recovery.

Patients must sleep with their head elevated and avoid any physical activity after nose surgery. Our patients return for an office visit five days after surgery for a checkup. We do place splints inside the nose that are removed at the second postoperative visit. Cast removal occurs six to eight days after nasal surgery. It takes another thirty days for a more complete recovery, with the entire results not fully evident for eight to twelve months.

Recovery and Follow-up Care

Your initial recovery will last several weeks, during which time you need to be aware of several issues that can impact your healing. Anticipate some swelling around the eyes for at least the first few days after surgery. It will diminish by the fifth to seventh day. Your doctor will give you a list of instructions that tell you, among other things, to keep your surgical dressings dry and elevate your head when you sleep. Keep the following issues in mind as well.

Discomfort

Sore noses and even headaches are not uncommon following nasal feminization. The discomfort that invariably occurs with a rhinoplasty normally only requires non-opiate pain medication. At home, the patients take oral medications, but the pain medications are usually only needed for four or five days. Although every person's reaction to pain is different, most patients need the drugs only occasionally, but particularly, when they go to bed.

Activity

Our patients begin minimal activity immediately, and walking is recommended right away. There should be no major or strenuous activity for a month. If you have a desk job, you can return to work in about ten to twelve days, but if your work is physically demanding, such as heavy construction, you will have to wait longer. Ask your surgeon about when you can return to work. Also, ask about strenuous exercise, because it can disrupt healing and damage your results.

Glasses

If you wear glasses, you will receive special instructions about protecting your nose throughout the initial healing. As long as your cast is on, you can wear your glasses. But after the cast comes off, you cannot let the frames rest on your nose even for a few seconds. You must keep the nasal pads that support your glasses from touching your skin for at least thirty days after cast removal. By placing a piece of tape around the bridge of the glasses, you can hang the frames from your forehead without hurting your nose, or hold the glasses up to see. If you don't wear contacts, before your rhinoplasty may be the time to try them; they pose no problems with this surgery.

Side Effects and Potential Complications of Nose Reshaping

As with other aspects of facial feminization, nasal feminization may have side effects. Your surgeon will share these potential side effects with you. The following are the problems you might anticipate.

Infections

Infections are usually not an issue with nasal feminization. There isn't a lot of space on the nose for blood to collect and form a hematoma that may get infected. We still put all our patients on antibiotics for approximately eight days after surgery to protect them against any infection.

Vasomotor Rhinitis (Nasal Dripping)

Patients with a history of deviated septum and enlarged turbinates who undergo surgery for major improvement of their airways are more prone to this embarrassing condition. *Vasomotor rhinitis* is a sudden and steady faucet-like dripping of the nose. This condition can start anytime, anywhere. Whether you are jogging or sitting still, your nose suddenly can begin to drip.

Some of our colleagues claim vasomotor rhinitis is a potential complication brought on by disturbing the frontal sinuses during forehead surgery. We don't believe this. Even though it may have several causes, we believe vasomotor rhinitis is most likely to occur with procedures that make significant airway improvements. Fortunately, nasal dripping usually can be controlled. We prescribe two pumps of antihistamine nasal spray per nostril, every eight hours, as necessary.

Nasal Bleeding and Other Issues

Nasal bleeding is rare with rhinoplasty, and major hemorrhaging is extremely rare. To ward off any major bleeding issues, however, your surgeon will tell you not to exercise enough to raise your blood pressure or pulse, or cause perspiration, during the first four weeks following nasal surgery. A *seroma*, a collection of fluid, can be an issue, even though it is very rare.

Hematomas, or small collections of blood, are also a possibility, but they, too, are rare. Small hematomas may need to be drained by aspiration, removing the fluid with a needle and syringe. You can usually stop any other minor bleeding by putting an ice pack on the back of the neck and elevating your head with several pillows.

Bruising

Most patients experience at least some bruising around the lower eyelids after nasal feminization surgery. It usually dissipates in two weeks or less. Some individuals, however, will have more extensive discoloration, particularly at the junction of the lower eyelids and the cheek. This discoloration can persist for up to ten weeks. Sometimes, a small amount of blood finds its way around the orbital rim and into the whites of your eyes, creating a mild scleral hemorrhage, which may also last even longer. Whatever the cause, the bruising eventually goes away.

Swelling

Most patients will experience nasal edema or swelling. Although it usually resolves itself in three to five weeks, some puffiness may benefit from nasal massage, a group of exercises that can bring it down even faster. Your surgeon will individualize these exercises for you.

Many patients complain after surgery that their airways feel obstructed. Even though the passages are wide open, the sensation is very real. It likely occurs because the mucosa or lining is producing less mucus than it had immediately prior to surgery. That dryness causes an increased airflow, which, in turn, can feel like an obstruction.

Spritzing the inside of the nose several times a day during the month after surgery with over-the-counter saline products usually helps. Also, be aware that the tip of the nose can become hard after nasal surgery and remain so for up to nineteen months. During that time, it will not be large, red, or swollen, so you don't have to fear looking like Rudolph. Eventually, it returns to normal.

We also will show you how to tape your nose after surgery. It is imperative that you continue to tape your nose for four weeks after surgery. This taping will reduce the amount of long-term edema that accumulates in the nose. It will lead to a pleasing result much earlier than if you don't tape the nose.

Septal Perforation

Some of our patients have a preexisting hole in their septum, the cartilage and thin bone structure that separates the nasal cavities. A *septal perforation* can be a complication of a previous nasal surgery or the result of trauma, cancer, other diseases, or cocaine use.

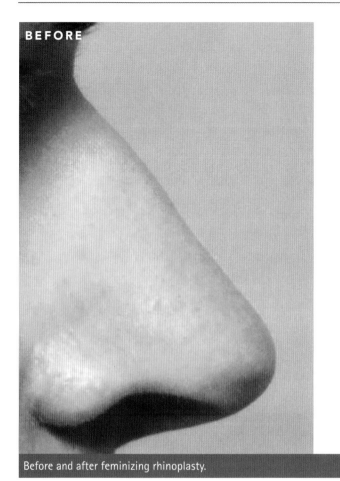 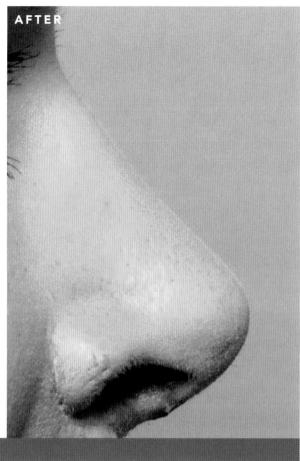

BEFORE

AFTER

Before and after feminizing rhinoplasty.

Septal perforation can cause bleeding, pain, breathing difficulties, and even a whistling sound when breathing. Although some perforations cannot be corrected, others, small or large, should be corrected with surgery if possible. We have repaired septal perforations up to 8 mm in diameter, usually using a "local" flap of tissue from the adjacent area to cover the hole. This problem can generally be resolved efficiently during the rhinoplasty.

Outcome of Nasal Feminization Surgery

Most transfeminine patients experience a vast improvement in their noses immediately after surgery. Beyond temporary swelling, particularly around the tip, they can see a new profile that is smaller, narrower, and generally more feminine than what was evident prior to the procedure. As the swelling decreases after the surgery, the nose looks even better. The final results, however, may not be apparent for several months or up to a year.

Commonly Asked Questions

Is there an age limit for nasal feminization surgery? No. We have operated on patients as old as eighty-eight. Obviously, patients need to be in good health, but older individuals can undergo successful nasal feminizations. On the other hand, for aesthetic purposes, we don't like to do this surgery on someone too young. We want to wait until the nose is mature, which is generally by age seventeen for girls and age nineteen for boys, to get the best outcome.

When we first started performing transfeminine nasal feminizations, our patients ranged in age from forty to fifty-five with an occasional thirty- or sixty-year-old. But because more openness exists these days about being transgender, we now see more patients in their twenties and even late teens.

Can this surgery be done with local anethesia? Yes, but general anesthesia is preferred. We want our patients to be completely relaxed during the procedure. It's much better for our patients to be completely unconscious during the surgery.

Is hospitalization necessary? Not always. Many rhinoplasties are performed on an outpatient basis when they are done alone. But we like to keep our patients overnight if this procedure is combined with other feminization surgeries. This approach makes recovery easier for patients.

Do you use implants in nasal surgery? We don't particularly like implants for the nose. When necessary, our strong preference is to transplant the patient's own bone or cartilage. Yet, if plastic implants are appropriate, we use them as well.

How does skin thickness affect the surgery and results? Skin thickness doesn't limit the surgeon's ability to do a nasal feminization, but it may affect the finer details. You cannot mold thicker skin in the same agile way you can mold thin skin.

How many times can you operate on a nose? The time between surgeries is important. We insist on at least a year between major surgeries; this allows the nose to heal properly. We've known plastic surgeons who've tried to fix a previous rhinoplasty before the swelling from the prior surgery had completely subsided, which only created problems; the physicians end up taking out more structure than necessary because the swelling interferes with their ability to make appropriate judgments.

There probably is a realistic limit as to how many rhinoplasties you can undergo. If your surgery is done well the first time, you shouldn't have to worry about revisions.

A Final Note

Refining your nose is an essential step in defining your new identity. Whether or not you're transfeminine, your nasal structure is perhaps the most important feature on your face. Because it's situated at the very center of everything, your nose influences facial harmony more than anything else. When the nose is proportional to your forehead, eyes, cheeks, and chin, it enhances your overall look. When it's misshapen, too large, or just a bad fit to your other features, your nose can make you feel terrible about your face.

As a transgender individual, your nose and how much attention it draws from others can take on additional unsettling significance. Your nose can either be a masculine signal of your past, or a feminine signal that you've truly moved on.

8

Lip Reshaping

IF YOU WANT TO LOOK your feminine best, lip surgery can be helpful. There are definite differences between men and women in how the mouth and lips look. For example, a woman's upper teeth are exposed more than a man's when she barely opens her lips. Yet, a man's lower teeth show more than a woman's when he opens his lips slightly. Having a robust *vermillion* (the red, fleshy outer bands of the lips) and a full vermillion border (the fine-line edge between the lips and the adjacent facial skin) are considered desirable feminine traits.

So how can you transform lips that are decidedly male into ones that are definitely female? This chapter explores how surgically shortening the height (or "vertical length" in medical terms) of your upper lip and augmenting the vermillion can dramatically change your mouth. You'll not only enjoy a more feminine smile, but also an upper lip projection that is curved and full. By making these changes, along with some changes to your lower lip, you'll have a look appropriate for your new gender.

Upper Lip Feminization

Surgeons can do several things to feminize your upper lip: First, your surgeon can reduce the height by shortening the space between the base of the nose and the top of the upper lip. Second, your surgeon can enhance the vermillion. This procedure is accomplished by inserting fat grafts, or, less commonly, dermal grafts, which are skin grafts taken from the *dermis,* or the lower structural layer of skin. We will discuss augmenting the vermillion in detail shortly, but first let's take a closer look at the topography of the upper lip and the way your surgeon shortens it.

Most of us think of our lips as the dark, reddish bands of vermillion surrounding the mouth. But your upper lip also involves the facial area directly under your nose. Granted, this space is not the same reddish color as the bands, but it tells other people a lot about your gender. The height of this space, as measured by the distance from the *sill,* or edge of the nostrils, down to the vermillion border of the lips is generally 3.2 to 6.4 mm greater in adult males than females.

UPPER LIP REDUCTION

BEFORE

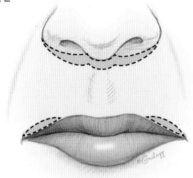

This illustration shows the surgical incisions used to lift the upper lip.

AFTER

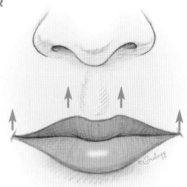

After surgery, the upper lip is shortened and more exposed.

Because of this difference, a woman's upper teeth show more than her male counterpart's when she opens her mouth slightly. This disparity becomes noticeable only as men age, beginning in their twenties. As the years pass, however, the lip droops far enough in males to eventually cover all the upper teeth.

Whatever your age, surgically shortening the height of your upper lip will help you appear more feminine and younger. The space between the base of the nose and the vermillion border largely determines upper lip height, so it makes sense for the surgeon to make the changes there.

Undergoing Upper Lip Height Reduction

Shortening the height of the upper lip consists of eliminating skin and underlying tissue between the vermillion and nose. Most lip reductions are performed under general anesthesia in a hospital in conjunction with other facial feminization procedures. But they can be completed as an independent outpatient surgery under local anesthesia as well. Out of the hundreds of lip height

reductions done in our practice, only twenty to thirty have been stand-alone procedures.

In either case, the upper lip is reduced vertically through an incision beneath the nasal sill—the little area or roll at the base of each nostril. If you do not have a sill, as occurs in some individuals, part of the incision will be placed in the floor of your nostril. By putting the incision in these natural creases, the resulting scar is nearly imperceptible. Your surgeon then removes the necessary small portion of skin and subcutaneous or underlying fatty tissue (sometimes including muscle). Closing the resulting gap has the effect of lifting or rolling up the upper lip, exposing a greater area for both tooth show and lipstick. It not only creates the appearance of added fullness to the upper lip's vermillion, but also uncovers more upper teeth.

Reducing the upper lip's height is a major gain for many patients who have thin upper lips. But, if these individuals do not want to increase the amount of their vermillion that shows, a different type of tissue removal is used, but it is performed at the same location. In either case, shortening the vertical height yields many benefits for transfeminine individuals. The upper teeth are exposed more fully while the lip projection increases because of the vermillion's new curvature. Together, these create a more feminine look.

Undergoing Vermillion Enhancement

Many transgender individuals want a fuller vermillion than that obtained through lip height shortening. That's not surprising because sexier, "pouty" lips are currently much in vogue among women. For many, reducing the height does not yield the full, robust look of a woman's lips. The lips are slightly fuller after undergoing a reduction, but they can still be fairly thin. Augmenting the vermillion, however, can produce nice, full lips. How is this done? By implanting your body's own fat. This is the best approach that we have seen for lip augmentation.

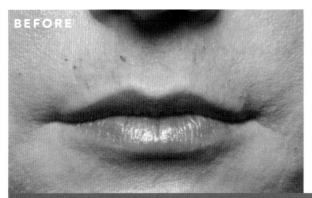
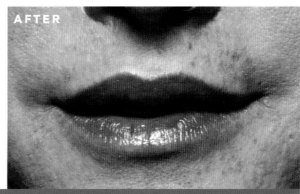

After upper lip lift with fat grafts to augment the lips. Notice the increased visibility of her upper teeth, which further feminize her appearance.

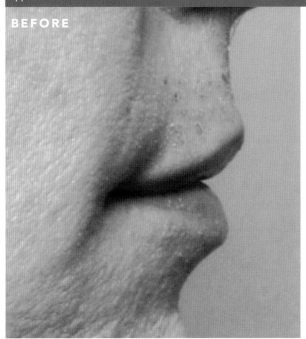
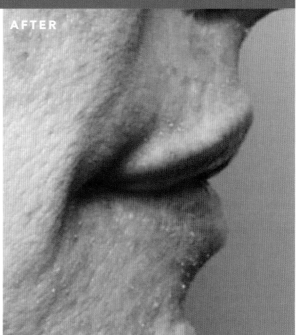

Fat grafting, consisting of connective tissue and fat, provides a safe, effective, and completely compatible option for augmenting the lip. The fat is harvested by suctioning areas of fat accumulation. We usually harvest the fat from the inner thighs.

In preparing the graft for transplant, your surgeon filters and purifies the fat. The fat is then injected with small blunt needles through multiple tiny puncture wounds around your mouth. There is no need to close these punctures—they heal without leaving any visible marks.

Fat grafting, performed by injection, uses tissue that comes directly from your body. When properly executed, augmenting your upper lip with your own fat tissue can look very good. However, the success of fat grafting can be highly dependent upon the surgeon's technique. We have developed techniques for selection and preparation of the donor fat cells, and our skill and technique in implanting the processed fat cells is providing patients with consistently excellent results.

There are now filtration processes that do not subject the fat to tremendous centrifugal forces. These forces tend to push the fat-derived *stromal vascular fraction (SVF)* cells to the bottom, and they are expelled prior to injection. Yet, fat-derived SVF cells are rich with nutrients and stem cells and should be retained. Our technique retains this material and contributes to our success.

Artificial Materials

Other techniques, such as threading Gore-Tex and other fiber-like materials through your lips or injecting the lips with silicone is often done to augment the vermillion. We do not recommend the thread approach because your upper lip will look stiff and not animate well. Liquid silicone injections are very unwise because they can cause a variety of problems, including swelling, redness, and lumpiness. Most importantly, silicone cannot be removed. There is no surgical technique available to take it out. Once it is in the body, it stays.

We have been able to improve the shape of upper lips previously injected with silicone by excising or removing inside portions of those lips. But the majority of the material stays in the body. The biggest worry for plastic surgeons is that the injection site might become infected. If you have not had silicone injections in your lips, please do not do it. We advise against it.

Hyaluronic Acid and Other Injectables

Your surgeon may suggest injecting a variety of other augmenting materials that are similar to those found in your body. Chief among them is a synthetic version of *hyaluronic acid*, the lubricating agent produced naturally to oil the joints and other connective tissue. Some of the products are better than others. Some may even last a year or longer. None of them, however, are permanent. The good news is that if the result is not satisfactory, the material will resorb in time, even though it could take up to eighteen months. The bad news is that if you have a favorable experience, you will need to have repeated injections.

When you have an unfavorable result with these injections, they can also be dissolved using another product called *hyaluronidase*. Sometimes, injections of normal saline may be useful as a trial run to determine whether one appreciates the look achieved when augmenting the lips or other areas. are considered desirable feminine traits with the upper lip procedure.

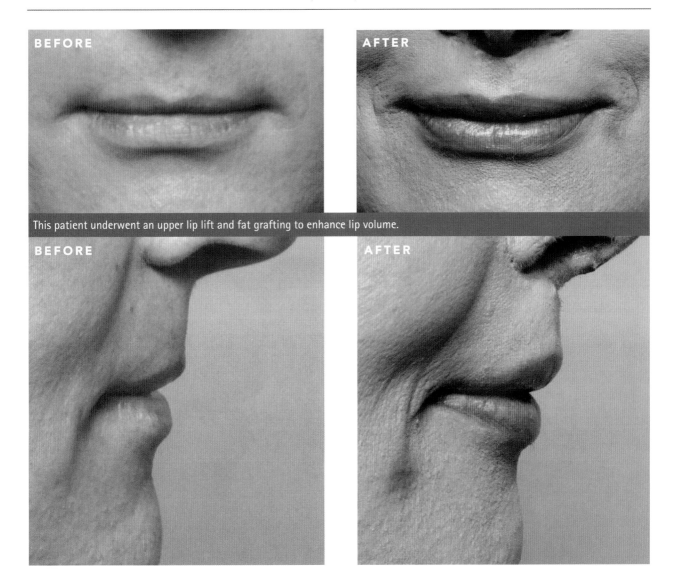

BEFORE AFTER

This patient underwent an upper lip lift and fat grafting to enhance lip volume.

BEFORE AFTER

Lower Lip Feminization

Your lower lip can also be a sign of your assigned gender. Unlike women whose upper teeth show when they talk or open their mouths, men, particularly older men, expose only their lower teeth. Why? Because their lower lips tend to be vertically short, just the opposite of their upper lips. That allows for the characteristic lower "tooth show" in males.

We know of no aesthetically pleasing way to vertically lengthen the lower lip. But a lower tooth exposure is usually corrected as a spin-off of another facial feminization technique called a *sliding genioplasty*. Discussed in chapter 9, the sliding genioplasty is used primarily to feminize the chin. How does that help cover your lower teeth?

During this procedure, the base of the chin is moved up to reduce the bony vertical height. With it comes the skin. That automatically raises the lower lip, which, in turn, improves coverage of the lower teeth. Because virtually

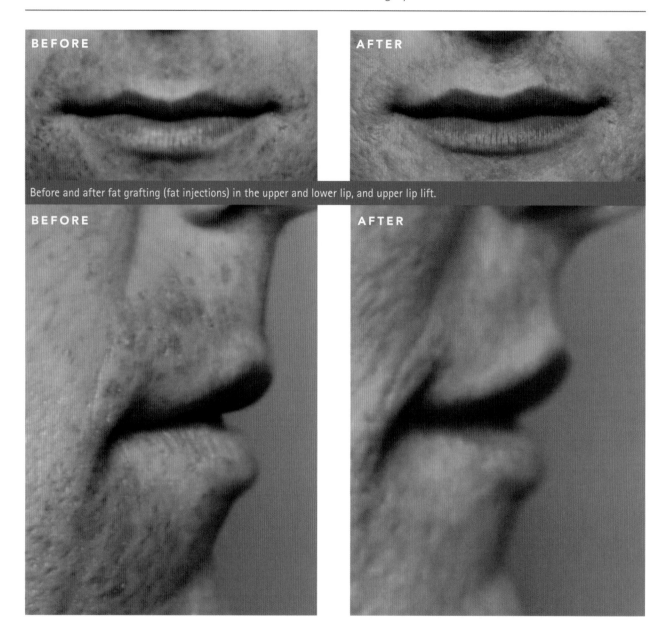

Before and after fat grafting (fat injections) in the upper and lower lip, and upper lip lift.

all transfeminine individuals need their chins reduced in vertical height in facial feminization, the amount of lower tooth exposure is generally corrected with this procedure. No further surgery is needed.

Upper and Lower Lip Vermillion Reductions

In the first part of this chapter, we discussed reducing the height of the upper lip. But there is another reduction procedure that your surgeon can perform. This one involves decreasing the fullness of both the upper and lower lip vermillion. Rarely do transgender individuals need their lips reduced rather than enhanced. But there are exceptions. If you have naturally generous lips due to your ethnicity or if you have had previous silicone injections, you may be interested in this option.

Most of the transgender individuals in our practice who have opted for lip reduction chose the procedure to correct the look left by past silicone injections. Unfortunately, silicone cannot be completely removed from the lip even though your surgeon can eliminate part of the affected tissue. Do not believe anyone who tells you that silicone can easily be removed. It cannot.

It is impossible for a surgeon to locate and remove all the tiny silicone spots after they have been embedded in your body. Silicone beads spread throughout the lip and are not easily found. We have also performed lip reductions for patients who have consulted with us after unsatisfactory results from overly aggressive fat grafting or lip fillers.

Your plastic surgeon can partially reduce the size of a silicone-enhanced lip using what's called a *lenticular-shaped excision*. Working through the moist mucosa of the vermillion, just inside the mouth, the surgeon removes a piece of tissue, curved on the sides and pointed on each end, just like a cross section of a telescopic lens. This shape allows for closing the incision nicely without a bundle of skin getting in the way on each end. A similar excision can be used to reduce the lip if it is just naturally large. In either case, we are very conservative as to what to take out. It is much easier to remove a bit more than to figure out how to put something back in.

Even after surgery, however, you will have residual silicone. Hopefully, it will never cause problems. Our biggest concern with this partial lip reduction is that the remaining silicone will become infected and not respond to antibiotic therapy. In addition, the residual silicone can lead to other issues such as chronic sinus drainage. Fortunately, we have never seen it in our silicone lip reduction patients.

REDUCING LIP FULLNESS

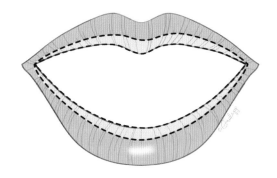

The dotted line shows the area of the upper and lower lip that can be removed to reduce the fullness of the lips.

Side Effects and Potential Complications of Lip Reshaping

Because the incisions for any lip procedure are in your mouth, they are closed with sutures that dissolve on their own. Your incision will not need to be bandaged nor will you need an antibiotic ointment. With any lip procedure you can expect a moderate amount of post-surgery swelling and bruising. Both are gone within several weeks, however. Hematomas have not been an issue with lip reshaping. If you are having a vertical height reduction, you might want to take specific note of the following additional side effects.

Numbness

Patients undergoing vertical height may experience varying levels of numbness depending on what type of technique is used. It is uncommon to have numbness after only removing skin and rolling the vermillion portion of the lip outward. Only four of our patients have reported a small area of numbness in the lips after surgery. The numbness lasted only three weeks for one person, two months for two others, and three months for the fourth individual. Normal sensation in all these patients returned. This numbness is very uncommon. However, in more aggressive lip-lifting procedures, in which it is necessary to remove muscle below the skin, more prolonged numbness may be experienced. Yet, we have still found this to be a temporary phenomenon.

Secondary Lengthening

Occasionally, a secondary procedure is performed to shorten the lip. Again, we do not consider this a major complication, but an event that rarely occurs. In our practice, about 3 percent of our transgender patients who have undergone a lip reduction required a second surgery because they experienced as much as a 5-mm increase in lip length, occurring in the first few months after their surgery. In examining the potential causes, we could find no consistent issues. The scars were excellent; they were not wide. The age, skin condition, and even lip habits provided no common denominator. Although secondary lengthening is rarely seen, minor skin excision revisions have been necessary to help correct this issue.

Outcome of Surgery

Lip-reshaping procedures are well-tolerated surgeries that yield attractive outcomes with some side effects but no significant complications. Of the more than 900 upper lip height reductions performed in our practice in transfeminine patients, the results have been uniformly pleasing. Whether patients undergo lip reduction under local or general anesthesia, they are happy with their new lip contours. As far as scars go, this procedure heals inconspicuously. We have seen only one scar complication, and it was caused when the patient failed to comply with instructions about her post-op activities.

In the transfeminine patients for whom we have enhanced the vermillion, the results have been pleasing and seemingly permanent. Although the inserted grafts are partially absorbed on rare occasions, this procedure has a 98 to 99 percent success rate, which is excellent by any medical standard. Our patients have been universally happy. A "fat" upper lip may be noticeable for a short while after surgery, but that resolves by itself. Most individuals usually see great results almost immediately. Patients who have undergone lower lip enhancements and lower or upper lip vermillion reductions, usually have a successful experience in our practice.

Commonly Asked Questions

How commonly do you perform lip augmentations? Fifty percent of our patients undergoing comprehensive feminization undergo fat grafting to the face. Of those patients, almost all receive augmentation of the lips. In our opinion, however, many more transfeminine individuals should have their lips and facial features accentuated through fat grafting. It is a relatively easy surgery from the patient's point of view. There have been no complications and the results look very good.

Do all male-to-female patients need an upper lip reduction? No. However, even in younger patients, we find that about 70 percent have an upper lip that is not proportional or similar to that of a similarly aged female. Certainly, younger patients (people in their teens, twenties, and possibly thirties) do not always need the procedure, but they may want to consider it in the future.

We do not know if *hormone replacement therapy (HRT)* will prevent the upper lip from lengthening. The great majority of older patients, however, usually benefit from an upper lip reduction. If you open your mouth, without smiling, and you do not see 3 to 4 mm of your upper teeth, then you probably should consider an upper lip reduction.

Do the lip incisions cause discomfort? Pain is generally not much of an issue with lip reshaping. Most surgeries produce some discomfort, but with this procedure little if any pain medication is necessary. Lip balm may help with dryness and make you feel more comfortable.

Do the scars cause any limitation of motion? The lip reduction scars in the mouth that result from reducing the vermillion fullness (to correct the results of silicone injections, for instance) may feel tight for a while. But they will soften with time and should not be a long-term issue. There seem to be no other problems from scarring.

Have keloid scars ever been a problem? We have never seen a keloid scar around the lip, nor have we heard reports of this problem. It is a place where such scars do not seem to occur, even in people who tend to form them.

I want the corners of my mouth moved up. They are low and make me look sad. Can this problem be fixed? Several procedures can be used to move up the corners slightly, but not to any great degree. It is not possible to raise the corners of your lips very much because of the many muscles meeting in the area. These muscles markedly limit what your surgeon can do to change the position of your mouth corners. However, the corner of mouth lift has been useful in many cases for rolling the red part of the lip out by the corner of the mouth and improving the aesthetics of the region.

Will I have numbness after upper lip lift/reduction procedure? This is occasionally possible, although it is temporary and tends to last approximately six months. This tends to occur with more aggressive maneuvers that involve removing a cuff of muscle around the upper lip to achieve a more profound reduction in upper lip length.

A Final Note

Reducing and reshaping your lips are important steps to consider in feminizing your face. Your surgeon can surgically reduce the vertical height of your upper lip, lengthen the apparent vertical height of your lower lip by a chin sliding genioplasty, and enhance the projection and fullness of both lips. Not everyone wants or needs all these procedures, but the right combination can produce an extremely satisfying facial feminization result. By changing your lip heights and vermillion, you can create a lip line that reflects your new gender.

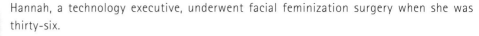

Hannah, a technology executive, underwent facial feminization surgery when she was thirty-six.

WHAT DID YOU HAVE DONE WITH DR. DESCHAMPS-BRALY?

I had my frontal sinus rebuilt. I believe I was the first case where he put a titanium plate over the nexus. I had my orbital rims reduced, eyebrow lift, very aggressive rhinoplasty, and upper lip lift. I already had a lot of hair loss, so he did not do a scalp advancement. He took a vertical 3-mm slice out of my chin and a horizontal 3-mm slice, then put everything back. He did a little bit of burring on the jaw. I had fat injections and a thyroid cartilage reduction.

WHERE DID FACIAL FEMINIZATION FIT IN YOUR TRANSITION?

After eleven years on Wall Street followed by two years of traveling the country by RV, I moved to California with the plan to transition there. Being older and having such a masculine face, the only way I knew it would work for me would be to get FFS. On day one of deciding to transition, I decided I was only going to do this if I did FFS. And luckily, I had the money to do it. I was on HRT for about a year before FFS. I was not really prepared to, but after my good results from FFS, my spouse said, "you have to go full-time immediately." Two weeks later, I donated all my masculine clothes, and that was it.

HOW DID YOU DECIDE ON DR. DESCHAMPS-BRALY?

I did a lot of research. I was obsessed with being happy with my results, but not with being conventionally attractive. A lot of the other surgeons don't seem that professional. Dr. D seems like the "extra-mile" professional. A lot of the other docs felt to me like a conveyor belt and didn't feel very personalized. I had originally thought I would have several consultations, but there was so much that turned me off about these other doctors. Exploring their sites and talking to other people, none of the others felt right. None of them felt like they were going to be aggressive enough. I also thought I should start with the one in my backyard. After my consultation with Dr. D, I felt like, "I can't wait for this now."

WHAT WAS THE CONSULTATION LIKE?

The technology that Dr. D uses is very impressive: the laser imaging of the skull, and his knowledge of the technical things. There's a level of artistry to it, but there's also a level of technology to help the artistry. Dr. D's demeanor also impressed me. He came across as a very intelligent, driven person who cares about what he does and takes pride in the results. That's the kind of person I am as well, so I felt very comfortable about that. I felt like he really did care about me as a patient, and that I wasn't just another case. It felt like there was going to be a lot of very individualized attention given, that he shows up and does his best every day. He also left no detail uncovered.

WHAT WAS SURGERY LIKE?

I was very nervous before the surgery, even though I made my peace with whatever would happen. I get anxious when I put my fate into the hands of other people, even though I had such a high level of trust with Dr. D. I took the prescribed sedative when I got into intrusive thought patterns.

My spouse at the time and two friends came with me. Because I am local, I was home the next day by 11 am. My release was delayed because it took awhile for me to urinate after the catheter came out. Physically, I felt very good even though I was tired, and I knew I had time off work. But emotionally, the way that I looked when I went out of the hospital that day did not make my brain or dysphoria very happy. I had my spouse cover all the mirrors at home, because I was a disaster, but every day I would be a little better. To me, the hardest part of the whole process was dealing with the emotions right after. You do this surgery to look a certain way, but there's this period where things get so much worse.

WHAT WAS YOUR RECOVERY LIKE?

I took about four weeks off, and I needed that not so much for the physical recovery, but for the emotional recovery and getting everything changed over to go full-time.

The swelling peaked in the first three days. I don't really recall my feelings when the bandages came off except that the discomfort was gone and I was one step closer to being healed. I was happy with the results at that point even. About three weeks later, I was able to look in the mirror and say, "Oh, that's you." At a month I felt very presentable. It took another three or four months for all the swelling to settle.

I had some numbness on the left side of my chin. Most sensation has come back, and if some hasn't, I have gotten used to it and don't notice. It never felt very noticeable to me, and it was worth the result. I had a little numbness on my scalp, but it's not bad. Sometimes when I eat ice cream, I feel it just below my nose instead of in my upper lip. When I'm walking outside and it's cold, my nose does run. Any side effects were fully worth it, because my quality of life has skyrocketed.

HOW HAS THIS CHANGED YOUR LIFE?

Although my facial dysphoria hasn't completely gone away—and it's unrealistic to expect it to fully go away—it's gone away tremendously. I just feel like me now. I look at old pictures of me, and I think, "Who is that?" Being deemed conventionally attractive by other people certainly has its privilege. I've gained that, and it's really wonderful.

My confidence has increased quite a bit. I felt my growth as a person was on hold before transition. I'm not super-depressed for the first time in my life. I'm growing as a person. And the world is seeing me and treating me very differently.

WHAT ADVICE DO YOU HAVE FOR OTHERS?

Try to do it once and do it right. Be sure you're making the right choice of surgeons. I am glad I chose a very aggressive set of procedures, because doing more later would have been a mistake.

The emotional part of the recovery isn't talked about a lot. In the first week, you do not look like what you want to look like, and there's a certain level of trust and patience that has to go into that, which can be very difficult.

Get yourself a good support network, including some people who have done it before. Very few people can relate to this experience.

You're going to get the surgery and look at yourself and say, "Ah! There's the me that I knew my whole life was there." But that's not the case for everyone else in your life who knew this old person you used to be. Looking dramatically different is something that other people don't handle quite as easily as you will. So, you have to have a lot of patience for people, because it can be difficult to get used to.

FFS, like all transitions, is a very scary and difficult thing to do. It's definitely the best thing I ever spent money on. The cliché is that it's brave, but a lot of people like me do this as a last resort, a live-or-die sort of thing. On day one of transition, you may not feel like a person who is going to be able to go through all these scary things and be confident and make the world accept you, but by the time you get done, you will be.

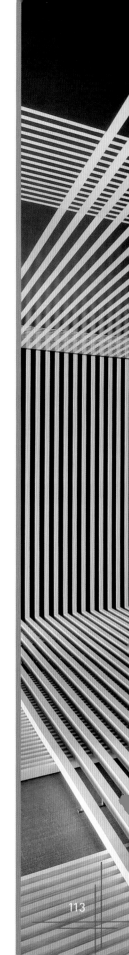

113

9

Chin Reshaping

THE CHIN IS AN EXTREMELY important feature in gender recognition. Marked differences between the sexes include the fact that chins are vertically longer and wider in men than in women. Is it possible that your chin already has the shortened height or narrow width of a female? Yes, but it is highly unlikely. Of the more than 3,500 transgender patients whom we have treated, advised, or met over the years, only twenty or thirty did not need a chin reshaping.

Think about that for a moment. About 99 percent of transgender patients need to have their chins reshaped.

Importance of Chin Reshaping

The chin is so different between the genders, that we highly recommend feminizing it for the great majority of transfeminine patients. The chin is the front portion of the mandible or lower jaw and the lowest point on the lower face. Anatomically, it's a triangular area where the two halves of the jaw fuse together. If you push on the mid-chin, you'll feel the *mental protuberance* or tip of the bone as well as the *mentalis muscles*, the paired muscle on each side of the chin midline. It supports and pushes up your lower lip.

A man's chin is generally 20 percent taller than a woman's chin. The dimensions are usually measured from the top of the lower incisor teeth to the bottom of the jawbone on a special skull radiograph called a *lateral cephalogram*. In addition, the male chin is wide, often with lateral or side prominences that add to its fullness. By contrast, female chins tend to be tapered or oval. Besides those gender differences, men and women can have other chin issues affecting the appearance of their lower jaw. Whether it's too high, too short, too wide, too prominent, too recessed, or too asymmetrical, the chin can be altered into a more acceptable shape. These differences must be corrected in facial feminization surgery. With a single chin reshaping procedure—the sliding genioplasty—a skilled plastic surgeon not only can feminize your look, but improve your appearance when viewed in profile and from the front.

Preoperative Evaluation

Prior to surgery your doctor should order a *panorex radiograph,* a panoramic or wide-angled

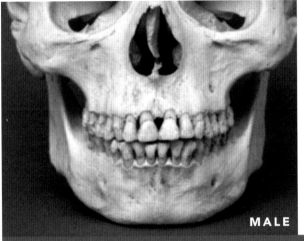
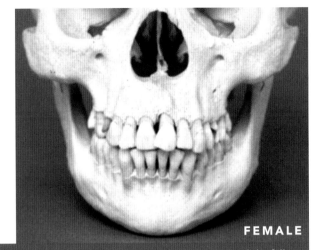

Compare the male chin, shown on the left, with the female chin on the right. Notice the differences in basic contour and the fullness on the sides of the male chin.

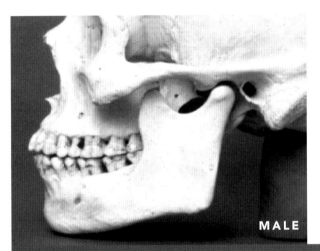
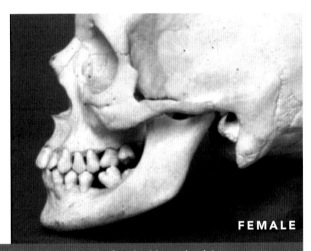

Notice the difference in vertical height of the chin in the male on the left, compared to the female chin on the right.

X-ray of your lower jaw, along with back-to-front and side cephalograms. These are radiographic images of your skull and facial structures. (If you ever had your teeth straightened, your orthodontist most assuredly obtained these same radiographs.) In addition, we obtain a CT scan of your facial bones as well as 3-D scans of your teeth. Taken together, these tests will help determine precisely what must be done during your sliding genioplasty.

The cephalometric measurements will be evaluated against various published male and female standards. Measurements were no doubt taken during your initial evaluation, but they aren't nearly as complete or precise as the ones linked to these radiographs. Your surgeon will also use the radiographs to evaluate other important markers, such as the location of important nerves. It is important for the surgeon to know the path of the *inferior alveolar nerve* of the lower jaw and the precise position of its branches—the

FEMINIZING THE CHIN

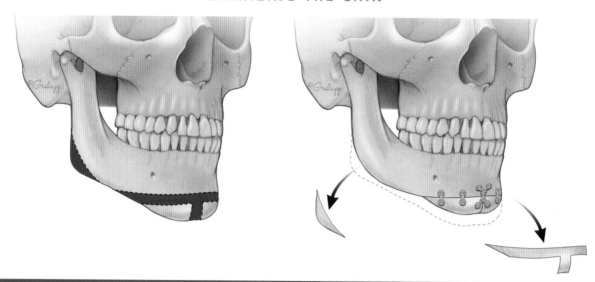

The area in purple above shows where bone is removed to feminize the jaw and chin. Tiny, custom-made titanium plates and screws are used to secure the revised chin.

right and left *mental nerves*—in relation to the root tips of your first and second bicuspid teeth. This will help your doctor avoid injuring them during surgery.

Your surgeon will also want to know the proximity of those nerves to the lower border of your mandible. Unlike motor nerves, which cause muscles to contract, the mental nerves are sensory nerves. They relay feeling from the lower jaw and chin area.

It is crucial for your surgeon to consider the relationship of your chin to your facial configuration, especially your profile. The front and back positions of the chin vary tremendously in attractive people, but they are always in balance with other facial areas. There are several techniques for placing the chin in proper relation to your other features.

Your surgeon may choose to measure the *nasal notch* of the nose (the juncture of the nose and the forehead) against the upper lip. Your

surgeon may use the *Frankfort Horizontal Line,* the line between the external ear canal and the top of the lower orbital or eye rim, drawing a right angle downward from it. Or, your surgeon might measure the midpoint of the nose through the upper lip to place the chin appropriately.

Whatever technique your surgeon relies on, the goal is to effectively produce the most feminine look possible. We use such measurements because they are necessary, and we also keep beauty and aesthetics in mind while developing our surgical plans. Ultimately, a successful outcome from this detailed planning requires one of the most essential surgical skills: good judgment. The most important consideration for any plastic surgeon is what looks aesthetically pleasing on you, the patient. Everything must be in sync.

Undergoing Chin Reshaping Surgery

A *sliding genioplasty* capitalizes on the fact that the chin can be modified in almost any desired position: forward, backward, upward,

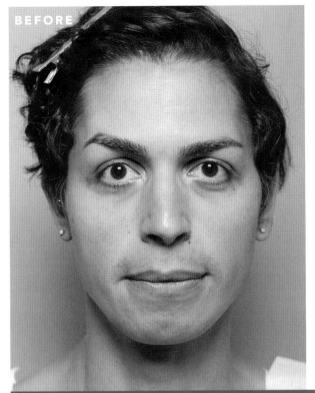

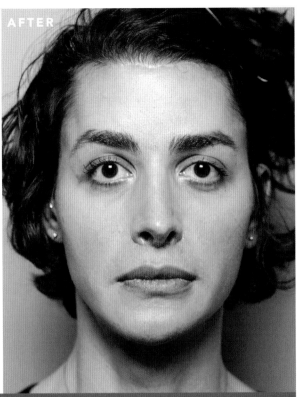

Chin reduction that included advancement and width and height reduction. Other procedures included: scalp advancement, brow lift, upper lip lift, thyroid cartilage reduction, rhinoplasty, and septoplasty—straightening of bone and cartilage between nostrils.

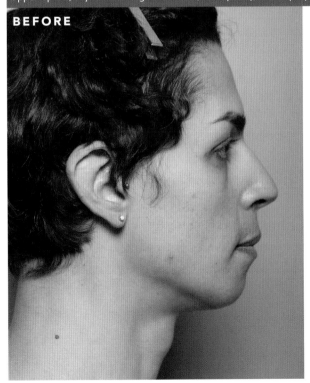

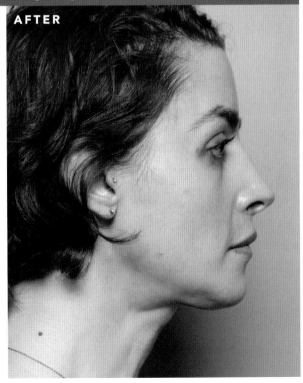

or downward. Hence the term *genio,* meaning chin, and *plasty,* meaning to mold. It involves cutting the jawbone (known as an *osteotomy*) in strategic locations and removing and/or repositioning segments to produce a more desirable appearance.

When we make major changes to the chin, we rely on the sliding genioplasty because it is superior to any other approach. Chin implants, by contrast, are specifically not recommended for this kind of correction. Instead of making the chin smaller, implants would make it larger.

Also, surface contouring (or burring down the excess bone) cannot safely or adequately feminize the chin. Contouring does nothing to reduce the chin's prominence or change its height. With surface contouring alone on any wide lateral or side chin prominence, you could also experience a major gouge in your skin because your bone will be permeated before the reduction is complete. Of the more than 2,000 chin feminizations performed in transfeminine patients in our practice, just twenty have only required surface work. Feminizing the masculine chin involves cutting and moving bone, not just removing bone, in nearly 100 percent of cases.

Unlike the vast majority of plastic surgeons, Dr. Deschamps-Braly is fully trained and experienced in orthognathic jaw surgery. A routine portion of his practice involves performing the complicated procedures required to move the upper and lower jaws of patients who have unsatisfactory overbites and underbites. Because of his comfort level with those complex jaw surgeries, the much simpler chin and jaw procedures involved in facial feminization surgery are, for him, rather routine.

So how does your surgeon use the sliding genioplasty to make fundamental changes during facial feminization? It begins with your initial evaluation. Let's take a closer look.

Reducing Vertical Height and Width

Because male chins are on average 20 percent vertically higher than female chins, reducing the height is important in feminizing the face. In more than 95 percent of the more than 2,000 sliding genioplasties we have performed during facial feminization, the patients needed a shorter chin.

Given the precise facial proportions your surgeon is looking to achieve, millimeters literally make a big difference. We have taken the chin height down as little as 2 mm and as much as 19 mm. Although the average is probably 9.5 mm, the amount removed varies from person to person.

During the procedure, the surgeon works through the inside of the mouth to eliminate any visible scars. The surgeon makes an initial incision on the lip side of the *labial sulcus,* the cavity between the lower teeth and lower lip. The entire chin, including the mental nerves near the first and second bicuspid teeth root tips, is exposed. From there, the surgeon reduces the height by first removing a horizontal piece of jawbone and then decreases the width by cutting out a vertical segment of the jawbone.

The remaining bone is then slid into place before securing it with titanium plates and screws. In a final step, the surgeon contours the lateral angles, eliminating the remaining fullness that makes the chin wider and more prominent in men. After reducing the vertical height of the chin, the lower border of the jaw will usually be lower in relation to the chin. In order to make sure there is a smooth contour from the jaw to

CHIN RESHAPING

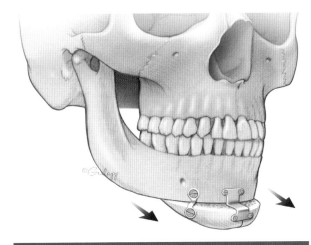

To advance a chin forward, a surgeon uses a sliding genioplasty, which is secured with custom plates and tiny screws.

the chin, the inferior border of the mandible will need to be removed as part of the treatment plan.

Your preoperative cephalograms will be used to determine precisely how much bone must be removed to reduce your chin's vertical height and position the chin prominence—or the lower-most tip of your face. Although we use the radiographs as a guide to excise bone for width reduction, we generally make this final decision in the operating room. Determining how much to contour your lateral prominences—those bulges protruding from the sides of most male jaws—can't be determined accurately from routine studies prior to surgery. This is when aesthetic judgment comes into play. In removing the side excesses, we depend on what we see and what looks right during the procedure to fashion the best contour.

As with jaw tapering, one of the most limiting factors to any chin surgery, particularly width reduction, is the basic shape of the *dental arch*. Whether it is tapered, oval, or square, the dental arch houses the roots of your teeth and mental nerve, the nerve that relays sensation

from the jaw area, and both must be protected. Your surgeon will achieve the most attractive, feminine look possible while respecting the anatomical limitations of your face.

Note: An implant cannot be used effectively to feminize or decrease the vertical height of a chin, because an implant is designed to add to the fullness of the face, rather than take something away.

Implants, especially those made of silicone, can also cause many problems. They can slide off center, rotate to an inappropriate angle, erode through the oral mucosa, and become infected. In short, they may have to be removed. They also can sit too high on the chin. What do we mean by that? If the bottom border of the implant rides up above the bottom border of the chin by several millimeters, the chin becomes unacceptably round. "Wrap-around" implants—prostheses that encompass the sides and the front of the chin—are a bit more stable. But they make the chin appear wider, which is not a desirable effect in feminizing the face. They are helpful in masculinizing the chin, but that will take you in the wrong direction.

Virtual Surgical Planning Techniques

Virtual planning techniques involve first "performing" the surgery on a CT scan. This is one reason for the necessity of having a CT scan. The level of detail is helpful not only for traditional planning, but is necessary if your doctor determines that virtual planning offers benefits. With virtual planning, we can produce surgical guides that are sterilized and taken to the operating room to ensure that the result we had on the CT is translated into real life.

Virtual planning is not used in every case. Yet, if certain details of the case call for it, the additional expense incurred in generating the guides and trying the surgery first in a virtual environment can be worth it.

Increasing Vertical Height

Although the chin height is excessive in most transgender individuals, about 2 percent of patients actually need their chin heights increased. To accomplish this task, the surgeon uses the same sliding genioplasty and osteotomy approach. After the bone is cut horizontally, however, the lower segment is repositioned downward to create a space for new bone growth.

The segments are then stabilized with plates and screws. Although the space will fill with blood immediately, scarring eventually replaces

it, followed over time by new bone. To help support the area temporarily, we insert a paste made from the patient's own blood. In addition, we insert the bone filler hydroxyapatite, made of sterile processed coral, and Avitene, a thickening and coagulating agent, into the space. The mixture becomes rock-hard solid in a few days, giving excellent support until the bone develops.

Advancing the Chin

Advancing a receding chin can have a dramatic effect on anyone's face, particularly a transfeminine individual. Moving your chin forward as little as 3.2 mm or as much as 15.9 mm not only markedly improves your profile, but can change your appearance so much that you look like a new person. At the same time, it can make

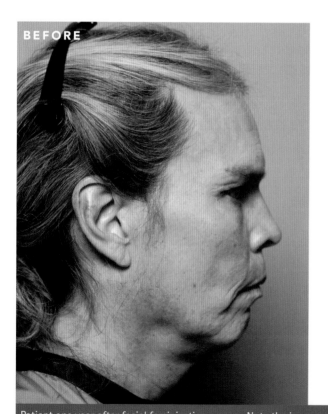 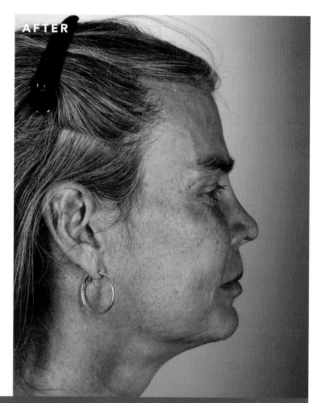

BEFORE AFTER

Patient one year after facial feminization surgery. Note the improved appearance of the jaw laxity after chin reshaping, which included an 8 mm forward movement. Other procedures included Type III forehead feminization with scalp advancement, rhinoplasty, jaw contouring, upper lip lift, and facial fat grafting.

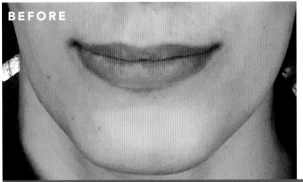
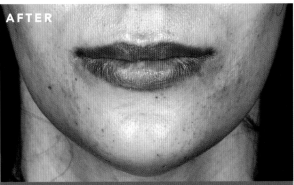

This patient underwent chin feminization to shorten the chin by 8 mm and reduce the width of the chin by 1 cm.

your neck look more attractive. The aesthetic result can be remarkable.

To advance the chin, we make the usual horizontal cut in the lower jaw and reduce the vertical excess as appropriate to the patient. Next, we slide the inferior or lower portion of the bone forward, anchoring it in front and back with specially shaped stabilizing plates. Because the plates are titanium, they do not cause problems. We can leave them in place, knowing that our patients will not feel them. The plates prevent possible bone absorption caused by tension on the surrounding tissues due to the surgical advancement.

We insist that individuals who need a larger advance more than 10 mm, wear a chin strap for six weeks post-surgery until the bone is completely healed. Why? The length and cantilever-type projection of the chin advancement is so far forward, that every movement of the *geniohyoids*, the jaw-opening muscles that are still attached, will pull the chin downward. The chin strap has been very successful in preventing a relapse, or the downward rotation of the prominent chin.

With an advancement of more than 6.4 mm, you might experience an unattractive deepening

of the groove, called the *sublabial sulcus*, between your lower lip and your chin. It can be treated during the surgery by placing a small amount of hydroxyapatite paste into the area as filler.

Some plastic surgeons have popularized the use of MEDPOR implants to realign the chin. However, this approach can result in various problems. Because the implant is inserted through an incision under the lower jaw, there is an obvious outside scar. Perhaps more important, MEDPOR causes a deepening of the groove between the lower lip and chin that is unattractive.

These complications are unnecessary given that plastic surgeons who are also trained in craniomaxillofacial surgery, can produce beautiful results without implants. By using a sliding genioplasty, your surgeon can not only correct your chin, but also take care of the groove in your mid-chin without putting you at risk for future problems. Also, the sliding genioplasty allows your doctor to produce much greater prominences than could be done with implants. Instead of widening the chin, this approach narrows it, which is what you want in facial feminization.

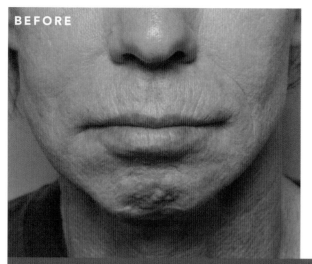

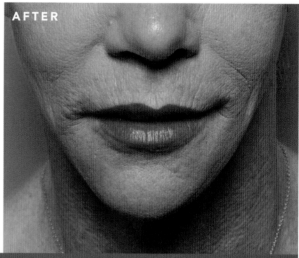

Before and after chin feminization that included width and height reduction. Procedure also included a significant chin advancement of approximately 15 mm. Later, the patient underwent a facelift and neck lift.

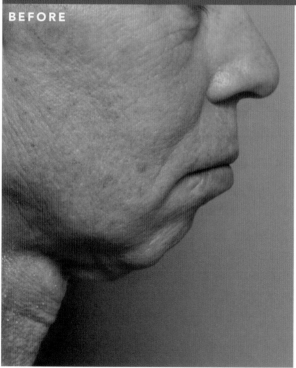

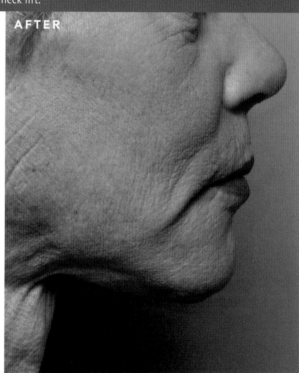

Setting Back the Chin

A standard sliding genioplasty technique can be used to reduce a prominent chin as well. After the bone cuts, the lower segments are repositioned back for better alignment with the remainder of the features.

Unfortunately, there is a limit to how far your surgeon can realistically set the bone back without affecting the *cervico-mental angle*, the soft tissue angle between the back of the lower jaw and the upper neck. A setback exceeding more than 5 mm will cause skin and underlying

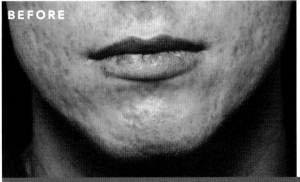 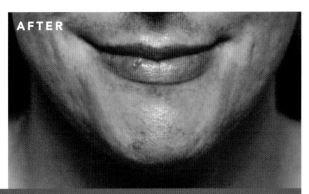

Photo on left is prior to chin feminization. Note the chin is off center, slightly lower on the right side. Photo on left is after chin feminization with chin advancement and width and height reduction.

tissue to accumulate between your chin and upper neck. As a result, you will not have a clean trim angle, and you may look like you have a fuller, aging neck. Even though your surgeon can recess the chin to meet your specifications, be aware of the potential problem of neck fullness. If it occurs, you may be headed for a face and neck lift to correct the problem. The final result may be worth the surgery, however, because you will have a better profile minus that overly prominent chin.

There is one last possible complication to consider. If your surgeon tries to reduce the chin prominence by contouring only the front of your jawbone, you can end up with a deformity called a *witch's chin*. This physical flaw

is described as a mass of unsightly fleshy tissue drooping from the front of the chin and an extremely prominent crease directly below it. Unfortunately, a witch's chin is difficult to correct because some of the soft tissue may end up back in front of the chin after the correction. A witch's chin is not a good look for any face, especially your newly feminized chin.

Correcting Asymmetries

The same basic sliding genioplasty technique can also be used to correct chin asymmetries. With this approach, your surgeon removes or repositions an asymmetrical segment of bone to correct the imbalance. Let's say, for instance, that the right side of your

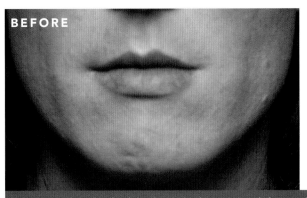 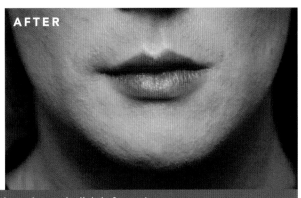

Before and after chin feminization to both narrow and shorten the chin, and move it slightly forward.

chin is lower than the left side. To accommodate the difference, the surgeon may need to reduce the right side by 10 mm and the left by only 6 mm, for instance. To do so, we make the upper cut of the bone even with the teeth and the other cut at an angle, lower on the right. We then remove the segment between the two cuts and bring up the remaining lower bone. In doing these maneuvers, we've corrected for the differences. The inferior or lower borders of the chin are now even.

Chin asymmetry is not a common problem, but it occurs occasionally, and when it does, it must be corrected. Patients are rarely aware that their chin is uneven. Usually, the surgeon points it out. Special mirrors and measuring devices can help identify asymmetry. The easiest way, however, is for your doctor to stand behind you and look down over your face from above as you sit. This vantage point allows your surgeon to see all sorts of asymmetries, from your cheeks to your chin, that are not obvious from the front.

Correcting Previous Surgeries

Over the years, we have revised many sliding genioplasties and chin implant operations done by other surgeons. Patients have come to us because the previous surgery had not resulted in a properly feminized chin or they had problems with the implant inserted by the first surgeon.

When a doctor has used the sliding genioplasty only to correct the front and back protrusion of the chin, without addressing the vertical height and width, that misses an important part of your chin feminization. A secondary surgery can address these issues. If you've had an implant, your doctor will remove it and perform a sliding genioplasty to correct

any bone erosion and properly feminize the chin. If you had a sliding genioplasty initially, your surgeon will perform another one to make up for any deficiencies.

One of the biggest challenges with a "redo" surgery are the preexisting screws and plates. Sometimes they can be removed with no problems. But in other cases, these genioplasties have healed so tightly, that they cannot be unscrewed and must be cut out with a reciprocating surgical saw. At times, this can leave residual metal in the bone. Yet, we have never been deterred from taking on or finishing a secondary procedure.

In fact, we've never had a case that we could not redo to achieve the desired effect. Of the more than 1,800 chin surgeries completed in our practice, about 9 percent have been secondary procedures. Regardless of the initial surgery, nearly all of these patients were happy with their new results.

After Your Chin Reshaping Surgery

As with every FFS, you will have to take very good care of your chin after the procedure. Your surgeon will want you to follow directions carefully because your success depends in large part on your attention to detail.

Recovery and Follow-up Care

You will leave the operating room with an elastic dressing on your chin that must stay in place for five days following surgery. The bandage prevents immediate postoperative bleeding. It also helps support the soft tissues during the early healing process. Because your sutures are biodegradable, they will go away on their own. In addition, you'll want to know more about the following.

Bone Healing

Bone healing in the lower jaw is somewhat different from healing in the long bones of the body. For instance, it may be difficult to find the exact location on a radiograph of a fracture in the femur or thigh bone years after it occurred. But on a facial radiograph, the line of the mandibular osteotomy may look like a "nonunion," or a fracture that has never healed completely. This appearance may last for many years, perhaps even forever, but has no impact on your jaw's function.

The plastic surgery literature has numerous descriptions of this phenomenon, so it is to be expected. Yet, an uninformed or poorly trained surgeon may think that a "break" on a radiograph of the lower jaw is a fracture or a genioplasty that hadn't healed correctly. Yet in fact, in these cases, the bone has healed beautifully. Since the introduction in the 1980s of internal plate and screw fixation, complications from sliding genioplasties have been nearly nonexistent. Of course, they must be performed properly to prevent nerve injury and relapse.

One of our patients who had surgery in San Francisco needed removal of an infected plate and screw three months after the surgery. The patient, rather than returning to San Francisco, wanted to have the hardware removed in London. The local physician was concerned about removing the plates, thinking that the visible linear shadow on the X-ray meant it wasn't healed. We suggested that the shadow on the image was not worrisome and the chin was found to be healed upon removal of the infected plates and screws.

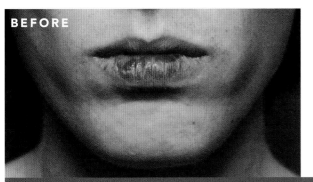
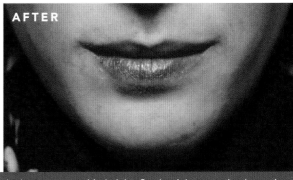

In photos on the left, note the fullness around the corners of the mouth, due to excess chin height. On the right, note the dramatic improvement from reducing the height and width of the chin.

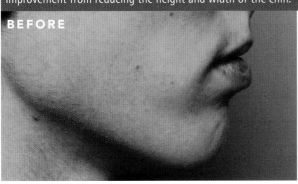
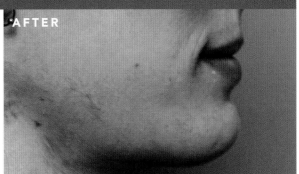

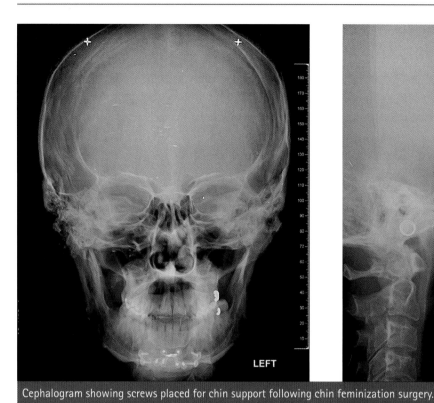
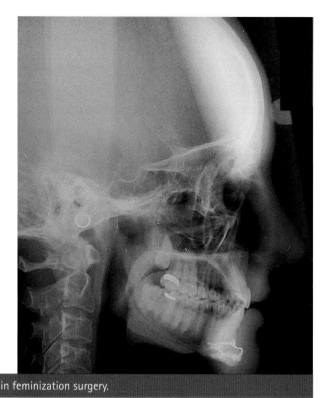

Cephalogram showing screws placed for chin support following chin feminization surgery.

Diet, Hygiene, and Activity

Because the incision for chin reshaping surgery is made just inside your lower lip, you must eat only soft (pureed or liquid) food for at least ten days. We warn our patients against biting into fresh fruits, fresh vegetables, or hard-crusted bread for at least three weeks. Soft flaky meats such as well-cooked fish, are generally fine to consume ten days after surgery. In addition, you must brush your teeth at least three times a day to keep your mouth free from infection-causing germs.

You should also keep your incisions as clean as possible. The usual guidelines about activities and physical exercise apply. Keep both at a minimum until your surgeon directs you otherwise. Also, make sure to sleep with your head elevated and keep your dressing dry when you bathe.

Side Effects and Potential Complications of Chin Reshaping

Chin reduction surgery is typically a very successful procedure. Patient complaints are virtually nonexistent. The pain medications used after surgery are very effective, even though many patients don't need them at all. As with other procedures, however, there are issues that you need to consider.

Swelling

After chin surgery, expect some swelling beneath the lower jaw, particularly in the area just behind the chin osteotomy. In some patients, swelling can be very significant, even though it eventually subsides. The swelling seems to be caused by trapped blood under the *periosteum* (the tough tissue lying immediately over the bone). Most of the edema will be gone in two to three weeks, but it may not vanish completely for up to six or even nine months.

Beginning three weeks after surgery, you will want to gently massage any swelling beneath the chin, using your fingertips, in a circular motion. To get the best results, we tell our patients to do it for one minute twenty times a day, rather than once a day for twenty minutes. Swelling connected to this procedure will generally subside.

Numbness

Many patients have numbness in the lip and mouth area that lasts for weeks, perhaps even months. This numbness is probably the result of pulling on the soft tissues during jaw tapering-angle reduction (See chapter 10), thus putting tension on the mental nerve. No matter where they are in your body, nerves do not "like" being tampered with; when they are injured, temporary numbness can result.

There are three things a surgeon can do to a nerve that may cause injury and/or numbness. The worst is cutting the nerve. The second and third are to "squish" the nerve or to stretch it; however, we must squish or stretch the nerve in order to avoid cutting the nerve. Thus, some of the numbness is expected for several months after the surgery. When your chin or lips are involved, any diminished sensation can cause other problems, such as drooling and difficulties with speech.

Through our own research in 1991, we devised a procedure in which we make the upper cut in the sliding genioplasty without injuring the mental nerve. Prior to developing this technique, 6 percent of our patients had experienced some permanent nerve-related damage after their chin surgery. But by making the cut about 6.35 mm below the mental nerve canal, slightly lower than we had done previously, we were able to avoid any issues with the nerve. That one little change made the difference between a lip with normal sensation and one that was partially or totally numb.

Since publishing our findings, we have completed more than 2,000 sliding genioplasties (in both transfeminine and other individuals). To the best of our knowledge, only four of these patients have suffered permanent complete numbness and one reported numbness on one half of the lip. This is a marked improvement over our results or those of any other surgeons prior to 1991.

Some of our patients have described numbness in a very narrow vertical strip, about 3 mm wide, down the middle of the lower lip and chin, sometimes involving the lower two or four incisor teeth. Neither our colleagues, who have experienced the same phenomena with their sliding genioplasty patients, nor we can explain this condition. Although you have a right and left mental nerve, you have no middle nerve where this numbness seems to occur. Although the source is a mystery, the lack of sensation seems to disappear in a few months.

Also, it is not uncommon to have a small area in the central part of the lower chin that has some prolonged or permanent numbness. Because of the location, patients have rarely found it bothersome, although they have brought it to our attention.

If you experience any numbness around the mouth area, be careful drinking hot liquids, such as coffee, tea, hot chocolate, so you don't burn your lips or tongue.

BEFORE

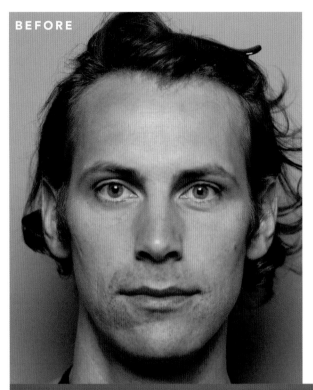

AFTER

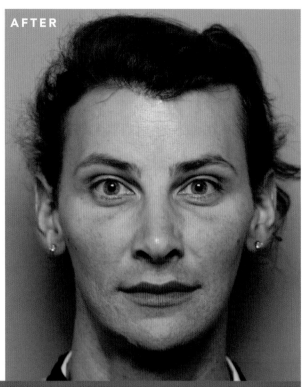

This patient underwent osseous genioplasty (chin contouring), reducing both the height and width of the chin by 1 cm and advancing the chin 4 mm. Other procedures included forehead feminization type III, scalp advancement, rhinoplasty, upper lip lift, panfacial fat grafting, and jaw contouring.

BEFORE

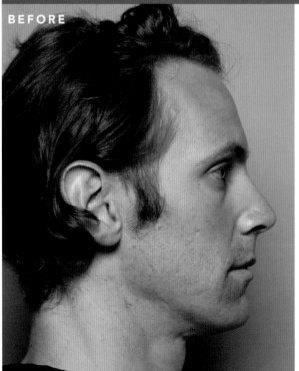

AFTER

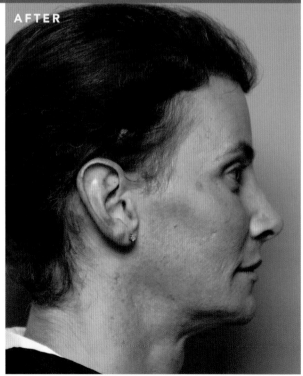

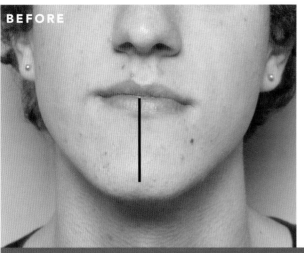

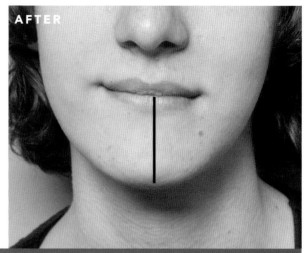

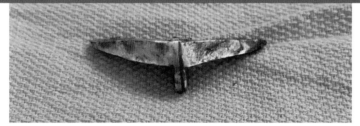

Before and after chin feminization. The black lines show a significant reduction in the height of the chin. The lower photo shows the chin bone segment that was removed.

Numbness and Drooling

Drooling or the sensation that you're drooling, occurs in some patients after chin-reshaping surgery. It occurs due to temporary numbness in the lip area. Food or liquid may pass over your lower lip and you won't feel it; then again, you may think something is dribbling out of your mouth when it is not. You may find yourself wanting to wipe your lips. Phantom or real, these sensations can be distracting. You needn't worry about a long-term effect, however. The lack of feeling usually resolves within a few months.

Numbness and Speech Difficulties

After surgery, your speech may seem slurred when you say certain words, such as "peanut butter," that require your lips to touch during enunciation. Although your lower lip is moving

perfectly, you may not feel it touching your upper lip because of the temporary numbness associated with this procedure. Although your brain might be telling you that you're not speaking properly, rest assured that you are. This will become apparent when the numbness wears off.

Major speech difficulties after a sliding genioplasty were at one time a real, yet extremely rare, risk. Occasionally, a patient would complain of difficulty enunciating words after their surgeries. The situation occurred when there was a significant (4.2-mm) vertical reduction to the chin. Removing the bone segment during the process seemed to affect the *genioglossus muscle*, the muscle that allows you to push the tongue forward as you move it between your upper and lower teeth. This muscle is important in speech.

We have been able to prevent this problem by stabilizing the base of the tongue muscle forward with a slowly degrading suture. Patients in our practice have not reported any major speech problems since we began using this approach years ago.

Outcome of Chin Reshaping Surgery

Chin feminization is one of the most exciting transformations in male-to-female individuals. It produces spectacular results in many patients. In others, the outcomes are more subtle, but still significant in their overall feminization process. In either case, the results are permanent and rarely require follow-up. Of the more than 2,000 transfeminine genioplasties performed in our practice, we have had to further reduce and taper the chin in fewer than ten patients, usually because of problems in the bone-healing process.

When we do have to revise a procedure, we may need to remove the front titanium fixation plate. In addition, we have moved two chins farther forward and one chin slightly back. The latter follow-up operation was necessary because we advanced it a little too far in the original surgery. To the best of our knowledge, no other modifications have been necessary in these patients.

To date, only two of our transfeminine patients have required any revisions to their chin. Dr. Deschamps-Braly has had three patients who required a hardware removal due to infection. One of these patients grew a type of bacteria on the screws that is found in hair follicles. That's why we recommend against manipulating hair follicles prior to or after surgery. In this case we removed some hair follicle cysts the patient had acquired from electrolysis, which was most likely the source of the bacteria.

One of the great additional benefits of a feminizing-sliding genioplasty, is its effect on tooth show. As discussed in chapter 8 on lip reshaping, adult males usually show their lower teeth, but not their upper teeth when opening their mouths slightly. Women, however, show their upper teeth, rather than their lower teeth when their mouths are slightly open. Unfortunately, there is no good method for vertically lengthening the lower lip to give males a more feminized and reduced lower tooth display. But the sliding genioplasty helps the surgeon accomplish that goal. By reducing the chin's vertical height, the doctor elevates the lower portion of the chin and, in so doing, brings the entire lower lip up with it.

As a result, lower tooth show is markedly reduced and may even be eliminated after a properly completed feminizing sliding genioplasty. The result is an overall feminizing effect on the lower jaw.

Commonly Asked Questions

Do you ever use silicone or high-density polyethylene MEDPOR implants for augmentation? No. The goal in facial feminization surgery is to reduce the size of the chin, and an implant only makes it larger. So, please, do not use them. Some surgeons use small implants to augment the front of the chin because they do not increase the width. But smaller implants especially tend to rotate, slide out of position, erode into the bone and *mucosa* or membrane, and get infected. Thus, your surgeon may be forced to remove the implants. Implants can also ride up on the chin rather than staying put at the lower position, resulting in an unusual rounded look.

Can a sliding genioplasty be done under local anesthesia? Yes, it can, but it is better to do the procedure under general anesthesia. After a colleague described the local anesthesia method many years ago, we performed two sliding genioplasties using his approach. The surgery was successful, and the results were good. Still, we found that the operation was too involved and messy to subject a patient to anything but general sedation.

What happens if my chin dressing gets very wet? If your dressing gets wet, it can cause severe skin injury. Much like fingers left in water for too long a time, the skin on the chin turns white and begins to break down. The skin is also prone to injury. You must keep your dressing dry. If it gets wet, it must be removed and replaced.

How quickly can I go back to work? The timeline for going back to work will depend on what you do for a living. If you work in front of other people, you may want to take ten to fourteen days off. If you work at home, you can return the next day, although you probably will want to ease up on your activities. Until your surgeon tells you otherwise, avoid any heavy lifting.

Although you will have some swelling, there's very little bruising with this procedure. Some people experience more obvious side effects, however, so don't be alarmed if you have more discoloration or swelling than you expected.

Does the hydroxyapatite paste you use to fill in for bone get infected? If so, how often? We have used hydroxyapatite more than 200 times, and of all our patients we have had only two

infections, both of which were resolved. That material heals beautifully in the mouth.

A Final Note

Most plastic surgeons try to feminize the chin by only performing lateral contouring. Why? Because they have never been trained properly in sliding genioplasty techniques. They do not know how to reduce the vertical height of a chin by taking out a segment of jawbone while protecting the mental nerve, for example. You may hear surgeons without this training say: "You're one of the lucky few. You have a very feminine vertical height. You don't need a vertical reduction. Some contouring on the sides of your chin is all you need." This is very rarely the case. Based on your chin, lower jaw, and lips, you most likely have a vertically high chin that would benefit from shortening.

Are there exceptions? Of course. Some of our patients have been feminized without having their chins vertically reduced or their widths decreased. But they make up a very small percentage of the more than 2,000 FFS chin surgeries completed in our practice on transfeminine patients. Well over 99 percent of them needed a height reduction. If a surgeon tells you that you only need jaw contouring to shorten or narrow your chin, ask to see the vertical height on your lateral cephalogram. Then ask the surgeon to explain the procedure that will be done. If you are not satisfied with the answers, seek a second opinion from someone well versed in sliding genioplasties.

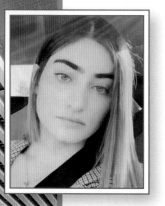

Camren is a health care executive who had facial feminization when she was twenty-three years old.

WHAT PROCEDURES DID YOU HAVE DONE?

I did the jaw, chin, nose, forehead, thyroid cartilage reduction, and the fat transfer at Dr. Deschamps-Braly's discretion, with the majority in the cheeks. The front of my hairline was in female range, so he just advanced the sides a little bit.

WHAT MADE YOU DECIDE TO HAVE THESE PROCEDURES?

First, to help relieve the gender dysphoria I was experiencing, and to be comfortable with myself, to have the inside match the outside. I was a stereotypical kind of handsome guy, so it was definitely the opposite of where I wanted to be. I saw that it would allow me to transition the way I wanted to transition, to achieve my personal goals and be my true self.

I had been on hormones for a year before FFS and was still presenting as a guy. Once I had FFS it was my plan to go full-time right after, so that's what I did. I was kind of alien/swollen-looking for about six weeks, and then it was, "Here's me!" The changes were definitely drastic post-surgery, so you're thrown into full-time even if you don't want to.

HOW DID YOU CHOOSE DR. DESCHAMPS-BRALY?

I did my own research on Dr. Douglas Ousterhout and Dr. Deschamps-Braly to understand their results, their training, their approaches to the surgery as well as the potential complications of the surgery. I really dove deep into their CVs, and that's when Dr. D really shined because of the craniofacial-maxillofacial approach. I had made my decision even before the consult. I thought Dr. D was the best, and obviously he was.

WHAT WAS THE CONSULTATION LIKE?

Before the consult I got X-rays done. Then from there, you go to the office. I remember Dr. D asking what I wanted and needed from him. That's when I put it back on him. I said, "I want whatever you think I need to get the best outcome." And then he went from there. I know he's a professional and, with anything, it's important to decide which route to go, but you should trust professionals at what they do. I didn't want to nitpick because I knew he knows his stuff, so I trusted him. And it worked out well.

WHAT WAS THE PROCEDURE LIKE?

The day before surgery, you go through Dr. D's presurgical routine in the packet. I felt a lot of excitement, and I was nervous, too. I didn't know what to expect. I took Valium and went to bed.

The next day I got up bright and early, and by then it was pure excitement. I really had no worries and wasn't scared. I remember falling asleep before the surgery, then waking up and feeling like my face got reconstructed. I had two drainage tubes and forehead pressure. It wasn't much pain, just discomfort. I was relieved it was done and I got through it. I thought of recovery as getting through hour by hour by focusing on fluids and walking around. I got the catheter out and Dr. D released me at 6:00 am to go back to the hotel.

I recommend having someone there to help. It's important for medication compliance and emotional support. My mom came with me and stayed the whole time. My dad and younger brother came for surgery and left after two days.

WHAT WAS RECOVERY LIKE?

At first my chin was quite numb, as well as the jawline and the forehead. The first six weeks I couldn't smile. It just wasn't connecting. I would say it was a good eighteen months before everything felt completely settled. I thought at twelve months I was fully recovered, but the jawline from twelve months to eighteen months reduced a bit more. The scalp is probably about 20 percent sensation loss. Other than that, the chin has come back fully, as has the jaw. But that was about six to twelve months before I got full feeling.

Logically, it made sense to me to wait until FFS to go out as myself. I didn't feel comfortable before that. I was in a position to do that. It's how I mapped it out in my head, and it was the preferred route, and it worked. Even though we've come a long way in acceptance, I wasn't comfortable then. I was somewhat androgynous looking because I was swollen and awkward. But I was suddenly gendered female almost overnight. It was like a switch flipped, and I was always gendered correctly.

I was in graduate school when I did it. That summer I did some online course work, and in the fall it was a completely new group. It was a bit nerve-racking because it's all these new experiences, but it was fine. It was nice to be me and be living my dream.

WHAT SURPRISED YOU ABOUT THE PROCEDURE?

In my head I thought it would be just like an overnight flip of a switch, and in a sense it was, because it was a massive reduction of my jaw and chin. But at the same time it was a healing process, and that is a journey. Looking back, it wasn't something overnight. It takes awhile to get there. Maybe I was being naive about that going in. The scar cream, the hair growing out, the swelling going down—all those factors take time. It's going to be a solid six months of dealing with those issues, and then it fades out.

Another surprise was having other women trust me more and the dynamic. It was affirming to feel in "the club." I'm my real self now, so people are able to get close to me. I'm being real, so people connect with that even more. When you can finally love yourself, you can have other people love you for your true self and not someone you're trying to portray.

WHAT ADVICE DO YOU HAVE FOR OTHERS?

I think this is the best decision they can make and the best investment of their money. It truly saved my life, so it's priceless. Dr. D finally allowed me to be me and be seen by the world as who I always wanted to be seen as. Everyone's different with their bodies and how they want to be seen and how they look.

Just go for it. Dr. D is the best at what he does, hands down. There's a drastic difference between him and second place. There are tons of different approaches a surgeon does during surgery. Dr. D is a brilliant surgeon, but he also has the aesthetic aspect to give what the patient wants. If you don't go to him the first time, you're going to go to him the second time to see him for a revision. So just go to him first and get the best.

HOW HAS THIS CHANGED YOUR LIFE?

I would rephrase that. I would say it saved my life. It gave me life. It gave me the opportunity to continue on and be me.

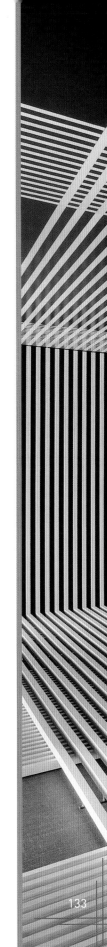

10

Lower Jaw Tapering–
Angle Reduction

TAPERING YOUR *MANDIBLE*, OR LOWER jaw, is an important step in facial feminization surgery. Women have considerably more tapered and narrower lower faces than men, partly due to differences in the lower jaw. Accommodating those differences is essential in transitioning from male to female. In this chapter, you will learn about the dissimilarities between the genders and the surgical maneuvers that can eliminate your jaw's masculinity. Making several select changes can markedly improve your feminine face.

Differences in Male and Female Jaws

To better understand how we will reshape the lower jaw, let's first examine its anatomy. If you were able to look down on your lower jaw from the roof of your mouth, you would see a horseshoe shape. At the midpoint is the chin. Curving back toward your molars are two bony segments, each known as a *horizontal ramus*. At the end of those segments are two pillars, each known as a *vertical* or *ascending ramus*. They

connect upright into the skull at the *temporomandibular joint* or *TMJ*, the jaw hinge.

The junction where the two jaw segments meet is called the *mandibular angle*. The *masseter muscle* is attached and located along the lateral back of the mandible at the angle. It's one of the major muscles of chewing.

Men have much wider, fuller, and outwardly bowed lower jaws than women, due to differences in their jaw structures. The *oblique line*, the bony ridge angling on the outside of the jawbone from the vertical pillars downward and forward toward the chin, is more pronounced in men. The masseter muscle is thicker, heavier, and stronger in males than in females, adding to the fullness of the jaw angle. Finally, the mandibular angle flares out farther at the side and extends farther back in men than women, which also adds to fullness.

Both the flaring and posterior fullness are a product of masseter muscle activity. Children born without this muscle have no angle at all. On the other hand, weight lifters, heavy gum

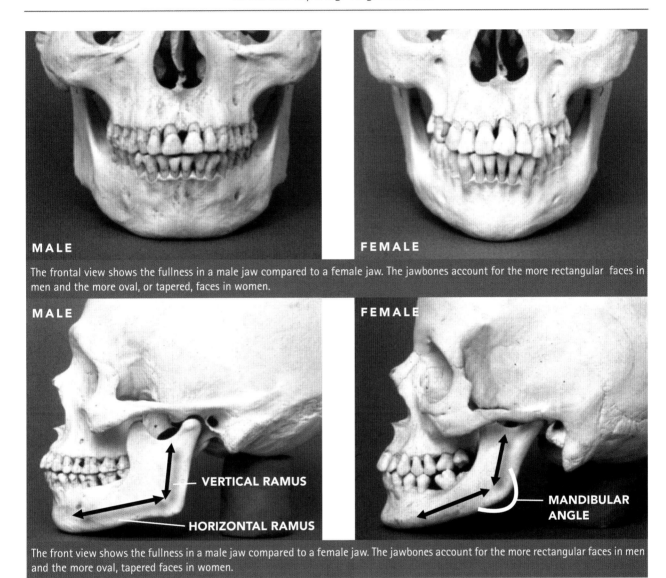

MALE

FEMALE

The frontal view shows the fullness in a male jaw compared to a female jaw. The jawbones account for the more rectangular faces in men and the more oval, or tapered, faces in women.

MALE

FEMALE

VERTICAL RAMUS

HORIZONTAL RAMUS

MANDIBULAR ANGLE

The front view shows the fullness in a male jaw compared to a female jaw. The jawbones account for the more rectangular faces in men and the more oval, tapered faces in women.

chewers, and people who grind their teeth have more lateral or side flaring. The reason for that is that stressing the bone causes the bone to grow. This is why resistance training is recommended for bone health in older individuals. Therefore, people who grind their teeth or chew gum will activate the masseter muscle and this often leads to bone growth in the area of the angle of the mandible. They also have more pronounced angles than other people.

Taken together, these features create the male's fuller, sometimes even rectangular, lower jaws. By contrast, women's jaws are tapered. Females have smaller muscles, slighter mandibular angles, and less broad mandibles than men. Their jaw-to-chin outline is either straight or gently curved inward at the angle. This produces a lower face contour that is narrower and softer than the sharper outline in a man. By appropriately reducing these three areas, your surgeon can transform the full, flaring, and relatively square

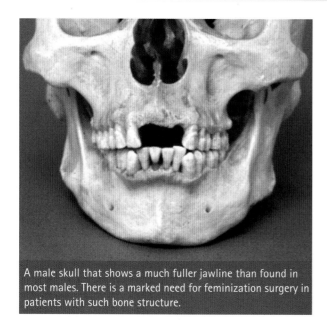

A male skull that shows a much fuller jawline than found in most males. There is a marked need for feminization surgery in patients with such bone structure.

jaw of your lower face. The result will be a jaw that is tapered with a much softer angle.

Undergoing Lower Jaw Tapering– Angle Reduction Surgery

In changing your mandible shape from male to female, your surgeon needs to accomplish three things. The surgeon must taper the bony ridge and lateral bowing of the jawline along the entire side of the lower jaw. The surgeon must reduce the angle where the vertical and horizontal segments of your lower jaw meet, and also remove the excess bulk from the overlying muscle.

Although this can be a stand-alone operation, it is usually accomplished in combination with other procedures. The operation itself takes approximately two hours, during which time your surgeon will perform the above maneuvers to completely transform your lower jaw.

Reducing the Oblique Line

The first step in tapering the jaw is to reduce both the side bowing of the *horizontal ramus*

(the prominence at the side of the jaw) and the oblique line, or bony ridge, between that area and your chin. This reduction is accomplished by burring the thick, hard outer cortical layer of the jawbone down to reach the central cancellous bone. In shaving the bone, we try to develop as much of a straight line as possible between the ascending ramus—the perpendicular back portion of the jaw—and the lateral or side of the chin.

We are limited in how much can be reduced by the nerves and vessels that supply blood and relay sensation from your lower lip, front teeth, and chin. Their position is one of two important limiting factors in this surgery. The other is the lateral or side roots of the teeth. We cannot disturb either of them. Through the years, however, we have become more aggressive in how much we will reduce the bone. Our patients have inspired us to reach further, resulting in increasingly better outcomes.

Reducing the Mandibular Angle

The second step is to reduce the angle of your jaw where the horizontal and vertical rami meet. For this, a portion of the bone must be trimmed. Using a special right-angle saw or a reciprocating saw, we work from under the masseter muscle. First, the side protrusion of the mandibular angle is burred away. We take a good deal of bone from the surface of this area before cutting off the lower and back portion of the angle itself.

The preoperative cephalograms, detailed radiographs of your skull, will determine just how much shaving is necessary to obtain the right contour. With rare exception, nearly every patient undergoing facial feminization surgery will require both jaw tapering and angle reduction. Of the more than 1,600 cases performed in

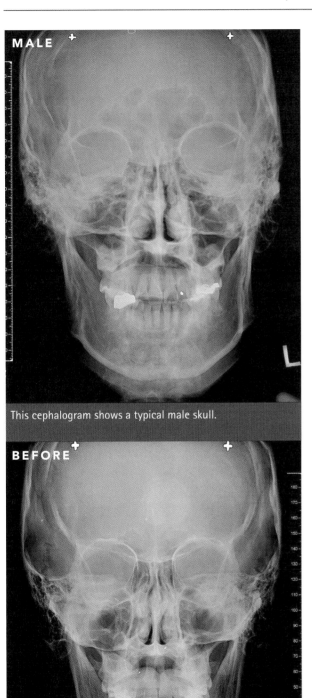

MALE

This cephalogram shows a typical male skull.

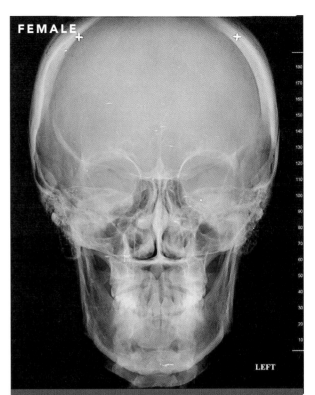

FEMALE

LEFT

Shown here is the skull of a typical female. Notice the differences in the angle of the jawbones.

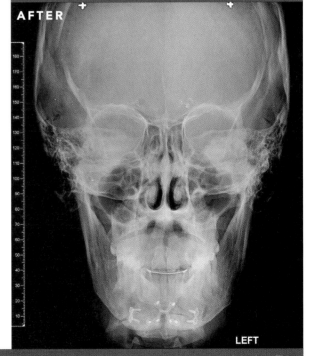

BEFORE

LEFT

AFTER

LEFT

Cephalogram of the same patient before and after lower jaw tapering and mandibular angle reduction at the corner of the jaw. The chin was also reshaped, reducing the height and width.

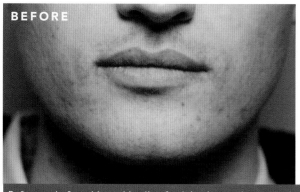
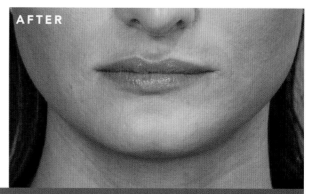

Before and after chin and jawline feminization to shorten and narrow the chin and contour the jawline.

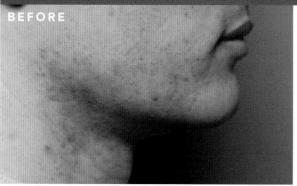
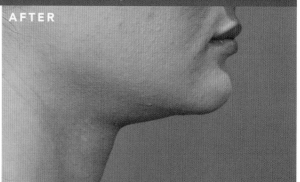

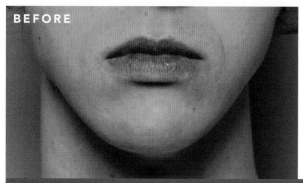
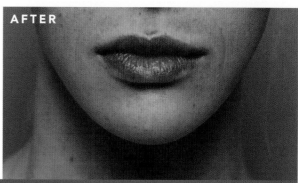

Before and after chin feminization, jaw tapering including gonial angle resection (angle of the jaw), and masseter muscle reduction (chewing muscle reduction).

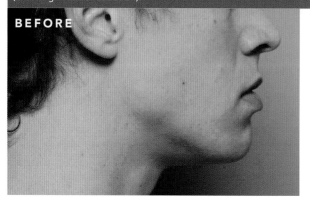
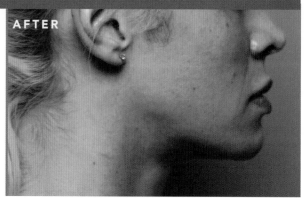

our practice, only one patient needed an angle reduction alone. All the other individuals benefited from both tapering the jaw and decreasing the angle. Dr. Deschamps-Braly has introduced a new technique to remove the angle of the mandible that is much faster and probably more accurate than the procedure we first used.

Reducing the Masseter Muscle

The third step is to reduce the masseter muscle by cutting and removing excess tissue from the *medial* or internal surface. This is the muscle area adjacent to the bone. By approaching from close to the bone, we can avoid damage to your *seventh cranial* or facial nerve. Again, the amount to be eliminated is determined by the evaluation prior to surgery. Not everyone needs a masseter muscle reduction.

Even in transgender individuals who need the procedure, the amount we remove varies according to each person's muscle mass and mandibular angle size. If we have taken off a large amount of the angle, we don't reduce the muscle by as much, because we know it will undergo significant atrophy from losing some of its function. But if the angle is small and the muscle is large, we take off much more. In either case, the amount removed accomplishes the goal.

After these maneuvers are complete, drains are placed on each side of the jaw inside the mouth. Then the incisions are completely closed. The drains are used to eliminate excess blood from the normal postoperative flow or "oozing" that occurs.

Are there factors that can limit your surgeon's ability to give you the ideal female tapered lower face? Yes. If the mandibular arch—the horseshoe-shaped curve of your lower jaw—is more round or rectangular rather than tapered, your surgeon may not be able to produce the same result as in an oval-shaped mandible. Why so? Your dental arch follows the same basic bony shape as your jaw, so your surgeon must work around the normal position of your teeth. Your surgeon cannot just uproot several teeth to accommodate a tapered look. Fortunately, square jaw shapes are quite rare. When it does occur, however, we can still give the patient a more feminine jaw. It just may not be the female ideal.

Correcting Asymmetry

Sometimes, patients have significant preoperative lower facial asymmetry. By varying the amount of reduction on each side, however, it often can be markedly improved. With the right adjustments, your lower jaw can look very balanced after the procedure, despite any initial asymmetry.

After Your Tapering and Angle Reduction Surgery

Jaw tapering and angle reduction surgery generally requires an overnight stay in the hospital, followed by a lengthy recovery until the lower jawbone heals completely into its new contour. During this time, you will need to pay close attention to your surgeon's instructions because there are many issues that can affect your final outcome.

Recovery and Follow-up Care

Recovery begins when you leave the operating room with a large bandage encircling your jaw and the top of your head. This dressing compresses the lateral soft tissue against the bone, reducing any postoperative bleeding. It also secures and supports the two vacuum drains placed in your mouth to eliminate any blood that might collect after surgery. Our nurses usually extract three to six tablespoons of blood from

BEFORE

AFTER

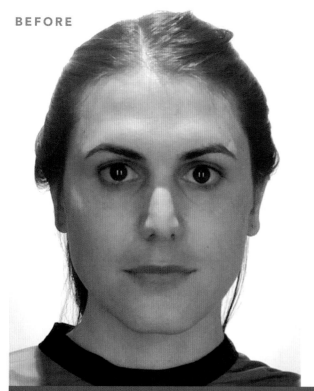

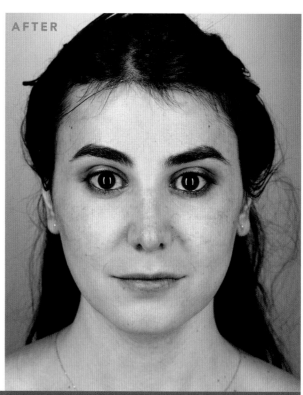

Before and after facial feminization surgery. Procedures included scalp advancement, Type III forehead feminization, open rhino/septoplasty, and jaw contouring. Patient also underwent height and width reduction of the chin.

BEFORE

AFTER

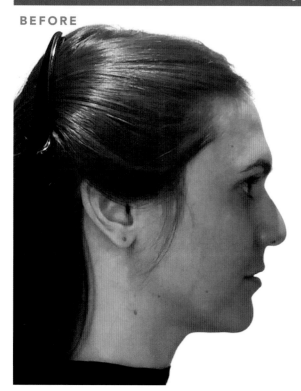

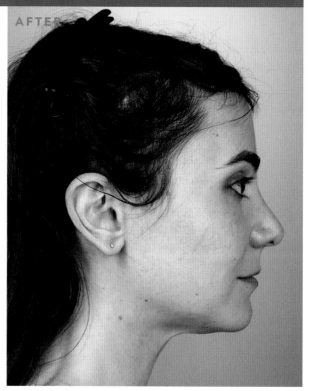

each side during the next fourteen hours. The drains are removed the morning after surgery, before you are released from the hospital. Your sutures will disintegrate in two to three weeks.

Diet, Oral Care, and Activities

Due to the oral incisions, you must be on a liquid diet for at least ten days following surgery and then a soft diet for six weeks after that. You must keep your mouth clean; brush your teeth at least three times a day and rinse with an antibiotic (Chlorhexidine) mouthwash. Do not use over-the-counter mouth rinses such as Listerine, as they can be caustic to your healing incisions.

The remainder of your recovery is consistent with other procedures. Sleep with your head elevated for two to three weeks and refrain from strenuous physical exertion. You can return to walking and your usual non-stressful activities and then build up slowly over the next two to three weeks. Avoid strenuous activity for at least a month after surgery, however.

Side Effects and Potential Complications of Lower Jaw Tapering

Most transfeminine patients tolerate jaw tapering surgery extremely well. Surprisingly, patients report little pain with these procedures. If they do have pain, medications usually work very well. Because discomfort is relative, it may not be an issue for you. Still, there are other potential problems with this procedure that you should be aware of before your operation. Although rare, the following are side effects that can occur.

Infections

Infections can occur with jaw-tapering surgery, but when they have occurred, they have involved electrolysis, waxing, or plucking hair. After a few of our transfeminine patients

developed infections along the lower jawbone, we finally determined that the one activity these people had in common was electrolysis. All of them had undergone hair removal around the time of their feminization surgery and suffered infections later. One patient even had to have her left cheek implant removed as a result.

Hair removal by electrolysis, plucking, or waxing can be extremely detrimental to your recovery. Although the needles used in electrolysis are sterile, the areas surrounding the hair follicle and adjacent sebaceous or oil gland are not sterile. With electrolysis, some bacteria may get into the bloodstream and collect at the site of a recent surgery, where they cause problems.

Note: We insist that you not have electrolysis, hair plucking, or waxing anywhere on your body from four weeks before surgery and up to three months post-surgery.

This problem doesn't seem to come up with other feminization procedures except for reshaping the cheeks. Laser hair removal, on the other hand, has not been a problem.

We also suggest that you shave with a single blade razor, and do not shave too closely for a period of a four weeks before surgery and three months afterward.

Close shaving has the potential to cause ingrown hairs and may be a source of infection at the time of surgery.

Nerve Injuries

Nerve damage can occur with mandibular tapering, and the biggest risk is to the facial nerve. This nerve sits in the soft tissue just to the side of the jaw. Because the rotating burr used to cut down the bone tends to grab nearby tissues, there is always the chance that the burr will catch on the nerve. In our surgeries,

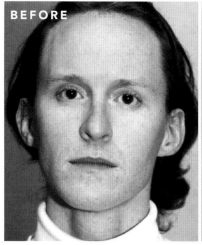
BEFORE

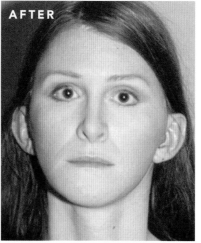
AFTER

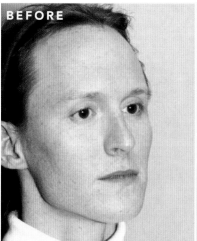
BEFORE

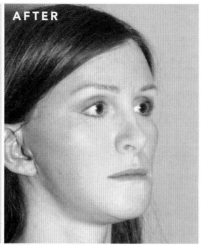
AFTER

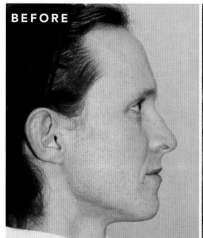
BEFORE

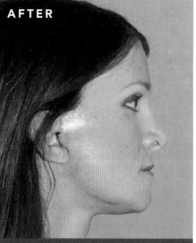
AFTER

On the left, before lower jaw tapering. On right, after lower jaw tapering. Other FFS procedures: scalp advancement, Type III forehead feminization, rhinoplasty, chin feminization, facelift, hair transplants, and thyroid cartilage reduction.

the facial nerve has never been injured. We are extremely cautious when working in this area. Surgeons must also avoid the mental nerve, the major sensory nerve. Yet, the facial nerve is the number one concern. Injuring it could cause partial facial paralysis.

Bleeding

Bleeding with jaw tapering surgery is usually not excessive, so it is not a major issue. Your surgeon will use special agents as necessary to control bleeding in the bone marrow area. The doctor must also avoid a large vein in the back of the jaw. If it is injured, bleeding can obscure the area in a fraction of a second. If a vein is nicked, the surgeon has to locate the nick quickly and clip, tie, or stitch it. Fortunately, most jaw-tapering patients have no major difficulties with bleeding.

Tight Scars

Some patients complain that the scars from their tapering surgery—inside the mouth along the side of the jaw—are very tight. They usually mention this issue around four to six months after the procedure. All wounds shrink after surgery; it's the nature of the healing process. But some individuals respond to healing with more vigorous wound contractions. We have never had to perform a scar release, a surgery to eliminate the constriction, because the problem normally goes away in a few additional months.

Mouth Opening Restriction

Some facial feminization surgeons believe that reducing the masseter muscle is dangerous. This is one of the muscles used for chewing. Some surgeons think the procedure could lead to a significant reduction in the opening of the mouth due to muscle scarring. However, we disagree. The technique to modify the muscle is not new. It has been performed since a Memphis surgeon introduced it in 1947, to correct enlarged and deformed muscles caused by *benign masseteric hypertrophy (BMH).* This is a developmental condition that results in excessive overgrowth of the masseter muscle.

Long before we developed FFS, we treated many individuals with BMH using this technique. None of those patients or any of our facial feminization patients developed limitations in opening their mouths fully, as long as they followed our postoperative instructions. After surgery, patients are prescribed jaw muscle–stretching exercises. If they do the exercises as instructed, they do not experience limited motion in their jaws. We have never seen this problem in our practice. No evidence suggests that surgical reduction of this muscle is dangerous. Craniofacial surgeons who do FFS, should know that the technique works and is safe.

Residual Fullness

Occasionally, patients complain that their jaws are still too full even after tapering. This problem usually occurs during postoperative healing. The body responds to the bony reduction made through the outer cortical layer and the cancellous bone by laying down a new thinner layer of hard cortical bone. In most patients this is not a dilemma, just part of the healing process. But in some individuals, the response to healing is so exaggerated, that the area becomes somewhat thick again, creating an excessive fullness. We have contoured this secondary fullness in a handful of patients, and it has not recurred.

Outcome of Lower Jaw–Tapering Surgery

The jaw tapering–angle reduction surgeries completed in our practice on transfeminine patients have produced pleasing results. Patients have experienced marked improvement in feminizing their faces. Do these individuals notice the results right away? No. In fact, we tell patients, "You probably will look worse before you look better." You can probably expect a significant amount of swelling and some bruising following surgery. It can take months for the final results to be apparent. It takes at least twelve to sixteen weeks after the swelling has subsided for the improved contour to become obvious.

Some patients say they see improvement five to six months later, sometimes even longer, although that is rare. These later changes occur primarily from partial masseter muscle atrophy. The muscle shrinks a small amount due to decreased function after the angle is reduced in size. Most patients are quite comfortable returning to work within two or three weeks after surgery when the swelling has subsided. Typically, the lower jaw heals more slowly than any other part of the surgery we perform.

Commonly Asked Questions

How important is jaw tapering to my feminine appearance? We think it is crucial, but this surgery is not absolutely necessary. It depends on the feminine appearance you want to achieve. All facial feminization procedures are elective, but this surgery is important to most transfeminine patients.

How painful is this surgery? Amazingly, the surgery does not usually cause much pain. Patients are often surprised at how little discomfort they experience. But remember, all pain is subjective. We anticipate our patient's pain and take steps in the operating room to mitigate swelling and subsequent pain. Dr. Deschamps-Braly has developed a unique anti-inflammatory pain management protocol that we have now fully adopted. It is so effective that very few of our patients require opioid (narcotic)-type pain medication. By not using opioid pain medications, our patients experience a significantly faster recovery. Why? Opioids slow the function of the gut, causing constipation; these drugs can also cause rebound pain when you're not using them. Opioids can also dull your thinking and decrease your motivation to walk and begin moderate exercise after surgery. In some cases, opioids can increase one's susceptibility to addiction.

Do I need antibiotics? Yes, antibiotics will be prescribed for you and should be taken after surgery. It is extremely important that you take the entire prescription to avoid infection.

I have a small mandibular angle. Can you augment it? Yes, we can, and we have increased the angle of the mandible in many patients. Yet, it is not a procedure we have performed frequently in transfeminine patients. In the few patients who required this procedure, previous surgeons removed too much bone at the angle, causing a marked concavity or depression in the side of the face. We restore the shape by inserting a prosthesis into that area.

This correction has been successful; our patients have been extremely happy. Never once have we needed to augment the mandible in a transfeminine individual who first underwent facial feminization in our practice.

A Final Note

Some transfeminine patients don't want the aesthetic results achieved with jaw tapering. These individuals have bought into the idea that a wide mandible is a very desirable look for a woman. This concept has been promoted by talent and modeling agencies vying for a different kind of eye-catching appearance. But facial feminization patients who don't have their jaws tapered or their angles reduced, may not appear feminine. Because the shape of the lower jaw can define a person's gender, jaw tapering–angle reduction is important for any transfeminine individual.

11

Thyroid Cartilage Reduction

FOR TRANS WOMEN, an Adam's apple is often a top surgical priority as they make a gender transition. Because this protrusion on your neck is so characteristic of masculinity, it may cause you great concern. Rest assured, however, your Adam's apple can be decreased in size. When performed by a skilled surgeon, a thyroid cartilage reduction can be accomplished without injuring your vocal cords. This procedure can significantly affect your transformation from masculine to feminine in a positive way.

The "Adam's Apple" in Men and Women

Your Adam's apple is known anatomically as the prominent forward part of the thyroid cartilage. This protrusion appears midway down your neck in front of your larynx, the part of your throat responsible for three separate functions: producing vocal sounds, preventing food from entering your air passages, and supporting your middle airway. Commonly known as your *voice box* because it houses your vocal cords, the *larynx* contains several areas of tough, fibrous connective tissue and several cartilages. The largest of these is the *thyroid cartilage*.

Your Adam's apple may be pronounced now that you have reached adulthood, but you probably didn't notice it during childhood. Only at puberty does the thyroid cartilage, and the rest of the larynx, begin growing, eventually becoming much larger in boys than in girls. Young men may need a bigger thyroid cartilage structure to support and protect the larger male larynx as it develops and produces a deeper voice.

Because a prominent thyroid cartilage is rarely found in women, it can detract significantly from your feminine identity. Reducing the size will enhance your appearance if you are changing genders. What does this part of your facial feminization surgery entail? Read on to learn more about thyroid cartilage reduction. Because an Adam's apple is an absolute giveaway to your assigned gender, it should be reduced. It is an important surgery for most transfeminine patients.

Undergoing a Thyroid Cartilage Reduction

Thyroid cartilage reduction can be performed alone or in combination with other procedures. About 3 percent of our transgender patients start

INCISION FOR THYROID CARTILAGE REDUCTION

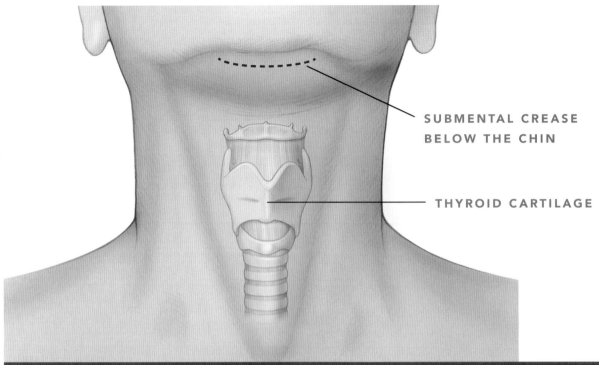

SUBMENTAL CREASE
BELOW THE CHIN

THYROID CARTILAGE

The preferred placement of the incision for thyroid cartilage reduction is in the submental crease below the chin. Some surgeons place the incision across the front of the lower neck; however, this approach leaves a visible scar. The structures shown above in gray are all cartilage.

with this surgery only, and some patients decide to stop with this procedure. If changing only an Adam's apple and nothing else, we perform the procedure using general anesthetic. When using local sedation, we have found that patients often follow instructions poorly and prefer to speak during the procedure. This can make it difficult for a surgeon to contour the cartilage.

We start the procedure now by marking the insertion of the vocal cords on the cartilage using a fiber-optic camera and placing a guiding wire in this area. This allows us to precisely identify where the cords are attached to the larynx. By using this method, we avoid altering or damaging the voice. We have had no issues with voice

deepening after surgery. We then inject the area with a numbing agent and vasoconstrictive agent that narrows the blood vessels. As a stand-alone procedure, this surgery takes less than one hour to perform from giving the anesthesia to closure of the incision.

If we are performing a thyroid cartilage reduction with other facial feminization surgeries, however, the thyroid cartilage reduction is usually done first. Then it becomes part of a much longer operation which is performed in a hospital under general anesthesia. Although the adding of other FFS procedures can make the surgery last up to eight hours, the segment for the thyroid cartilage takes only about thirty minutes.

ACCESS TO THYROID CARTILAGE

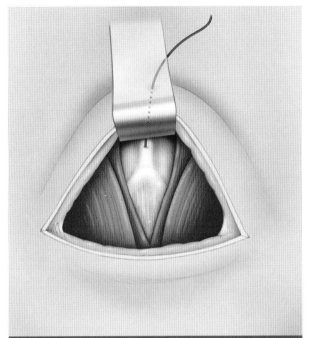

This illustration shows the access to the thyroid cartilage after an incision is made under chin. The gray area in between the two muscles which are shown in red is the thyroid cartilage.

Submental Approach

We use a *submental approach* to perform thyroid cartilage reductions, because it produces a more aesthetic result compared to an *anterior* (front) neck incision. The submental approach, however, does require more skill.

An incision that neither you nor the rest of the world can see, is the biggest plus to the submental thyroid cartilage reduction approach. We first expose the tissue through a 2.5-cm incision in the *submental region,* the area under the lower jaw between the chin and the *submental cervical angle* (top of the neck). With this technique, we can approach the Adam's apple without leaving evidence of the surgery on the front of the neck. The actual reduction is accomplished with a tool called a *rongeur.* With

it, we remove small pieces of the exposed structure until we achieve the right contour.

Although a thyroid cartilage reduction is often referred to as a *tracheal shave,* this is a misnomer. The surgery is performed on the thyroid cartilage, not the trachea. Although the two structures are close to each other, this procedure avoids your airway. A small bite-by-bite reduction, not a shave, is used to achieve an appropriate contour.

To be successful, a surgeon must know what to reduce and when to stop in order to avoid injury to the airway or voice box. This task becomes more challenging as people age (sometimes as young as thirty) because their thyroid cartilages can harden *(ossify)* into bone. *Ossification* is a normal process that occurs with aging, but an abundance of hardening can make reducing the thyroid cartilage structure more difficult. A surgeon must take extremely small bites with the rongeur to avoid inadvertently fracturing the thyroid cartilage.

Entering the area from beneath the lower jaw not only decreases the risk of injuring the recurrent laryngeal nerve, but produces a more aesthetic result. With this approach, we also completely avoid the possibility of creating a retracting scar that pulls up under the skin every time you swallow. Using this procedure, a submental scar is virtually imperceptible to the public, and even close friends, unless someone inspects the underside of your chin.

Cartilage Reduction and Voice Box Surgery

Is there any time when a neck incision rather than a submental approach might be appropriate? When performing a *cricoid-thyroid approximation* (voice surgery), your surgeon probably will choose to enter from the neck.

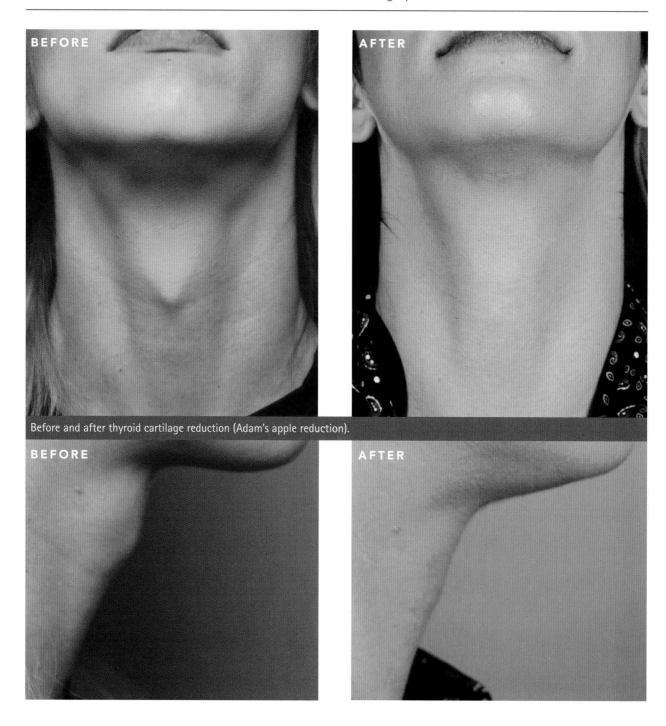

Before and after thyroid cartilage reduction (Adam's apple reduction).

This procedure is designed to modify your voice pitch by suturing the thyroid cartilage to the *cricoid cartilage*, a ring of cartilage in the larynx that connects the thyroid cartilage and trachea. Doing so limits the extent to which the vocal cords can relax, thus preventing the voice from dropping too low.

Some surgeons are doing a different version of this surgery through an *intraoral* (through the mouth) route and thus avoid a scar altogether.

We cannot comment on the long-term efficacy of this approach. A few select surgeons can produce good results, but most often, the outcome is disappointing for facial feminization patients.

We do not perform cricoid-thyroid approximations, but caution patients who are interested in the procedure to exercise good judgment when selecting a surgeon. Besides checking the doctor's credentials and experience, make sure you talk to several former patients. You will want to know, for instance, how long ago they had the procedure and the nature of the results. You should also ask about the surgeon's rate of successful outcomes.

Make sure you understand the surgeon's track record with problems, too. Ask about bad results, no results at all, and what the surgeon can do to address complications. Remember also that cricoid-thyroid approximations are not a panacea for feminizing the voice. The best and most consistent way to do that, in our opinion, is still with speech therapy and a lot of practice. And don't forget that this surgery causes a neck scar that can be very obvious.

Revision of a Bad and/or Retracting Neck Scar

Anterior Neck Scar

A bad and/or wide anterior neck scar or a scar that retracts when you swallow can be fixed. Your surgeon will complete the revision either alone under local anesthesia or under general anesthesia at the time of other facial feminization surgeries. The procedure is generally not very painful postoperatively. You will still have a scar, because that is nature's way of healing. Hopefully, it won't be very noticeable. If your surgeon places a substantial layer of fat between the skin and the thyroid cartilage, retraction should no longer be a problem. Postoperative massaging of the scar in a circular motion, using the fingertips, will help in the healing process.

Note: If your surgeon proposes to use a frontal neck incision to perform your thyroid cartilage reduction, you should stop and seriously consider finding another surgeon. That surgical technique is now seriously antiquated, and the risk of a clearly visible scar, especially while swallowing, is substantial.

After Your Surgery

Most people tolerate thyroid cartilage reduction surgery well. Whether you are undergoing it along with other facial feminization procedures, or by itself, you will be asked to follow many of the same guidelines that apply to other facial feminization procedures.

Recovery and Follow-up Care

Patients undergoing a thyroid cartilage reduction along with other feminization procedures usually stay in the hospital one night. If you are having no other procedures, however, you can go home the same day. In either case, no drains or major dressings are used. Patients leave the operating room with little more than a small gauze bandage covering their incision. You can use your voice immediately, but you should not lift or do other physical activities for several weeks. Straining might trigger bleeding. This bleeding can be severe or may just cause bruising and delayed healing. Although your situation will not be life threatening, you could experience significant swelling. We like to see our patients on the fifth day after surgery for follow-up and to remove the skin sutures, which are placed in two layers of the skin.

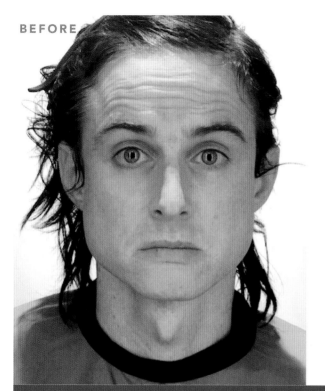

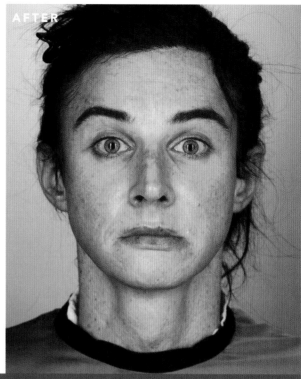

Before and after forehead feminization, chin and jawline contouring with masseter muscle reduction (chewing muscle reduction), thyroid cartilage reduction (Adam's apple reduction), and feminizing rhinoplasty.

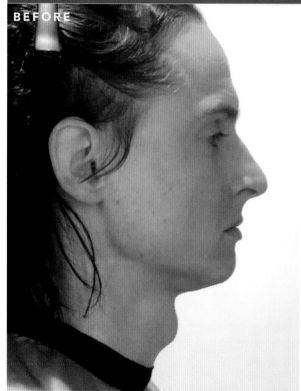

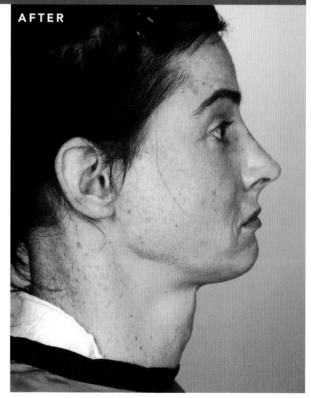

Side Effects and Potential Complications of Thyroid Cartilage Surgery

Following cartilage reduction surgery, patients experience very little swelling and bruising. Any bruising usually goes away in a few days. There is little or no pain. Some patients report a sore throat or hoarseness, although these issues usually last for only two to three days. Infections, *hematomas* (blood pooling under the skin), and *seromas* (pockets of fluid also under the skin) are a possibility with any surgery, but they are rare with this one. In fact, depending on your individual tolerance, you may experience no pain or negative after effects from this surgery.

Complications linked to thyroid cartilage reduction are rare. A few reported cases of long-term problems have been linked to this surgery, but none of our patients have experienced issues such as injuries to the vocal cords, the nerves that control them, or the thyroid cartilage itself. One of the advantages of approaching the thyroid cartilage from under the chin, is that we completely avoid the recurrent laryngeal nerves. Also, by conservatively removing cartilage, we do not touch the vocal cords.

Approximately 35 percent of our patients report a temporary lowering of their voices and narrowing of their vocal ranges (they cannot go as high or low as previously). Yet, this usually resolves itself in three to four days, much like a cold or sore throat. The likely cause of the voice issues is swelling at the site. To date, only two patients have experienced a vocal change or hoarseness that lasted for one to several months or more. All of our patients can speak during their recovery, and all have had a normal voice over time.

Outcome of Surgery

By removing your prominent Adam's apple, thyroid cartilage reduction surgery eliminates the most obvious facial evidence of your assigned gender. This procedure requires a skilled surgeon who knows the thyroid-trachea mechanism well. It yields some of the most satisfying outcomes in facial feminization. You will see the results immediately because the protrusion is gone.

Unfortunately, not all people exhibit the same neck anatomy. Some individuals have a very prominent thyroid-tracheal mechanism; therefore, even a well-executed reduction might not yield the optimal result. We can give you a nice new contour, but the position of your esophagus and the backbone behind the cartilage may prevent moving the whole structure back far enough to achieve the look you'd like.

Still, the surgery can produce a significantly more feminine neck contour than you currently have. The hundreds of reductions completed in our practice have yielded consistent and pleasing results. So, no matter the size, a thyroid cartilage reduction can eliminate one of the most obvious facial signs of your assigned gender—your Adam's apple.

Commonly Asked Questions

My surgeon says that the only way to reduce my Adam's apple is with a front-of-the-neck incision. Is that true? No. In fact, just the opposite is true. It is much safer to enter through the submental area, the area behind the chin, than cutting on the front of the neck. The resulting scar is not only less apparent, but also never retracts or rides up when you swallow. After years of performing this procedure through the submental area, we are convinced that it's much safer and more effective than any other approach.

Is there an age limit on this surgery? No, we have performed this procedure even on people in their seventies. They have experienced no problems.

Can this surgery be performed under local anesthesia? Yes, we can perform thyroid cartilage reductions as an isolated procedure with just local anesthesia. Yet, we still recommend general anesthesia for the best results and patient comfort. The entire procedure, from entering the operating room to leaving for recovery, usually takes less than sixty minutes.

Have you ever had to redo a thyroid cartilage reduction? Yes. We have gone back to further reduce an area of prominence in maybe eight to ten cases where we originally thought we had adequately addressed the Adam's apple during the original surgery. Although it is inconvenient, our patients have been happy with the final result.

Can permanent voice loss occur after a thyroid cartilage reduction? Yes, but fortunately, neither of us have ever experienced it with any of our patients. However, it has been reported in the medical literature.

I have been told that it would be too dangerous to place the incision in the submental area, because my neck is too long. Is that true? We have operated successfully on many patients with long necks using the submental technique. Please understand that surgeons who do not know how to do this surgery properly may try to convince you that thyroid cartilage reduction should be done with an incision in your neck. You should have the procedure through a submental incision under and behind the chin where it is much less detectable, if at all.

Can additional reduction be performed after voice surgery? Yes, although we don't exactly know the risk for voice change when thyroid cartilage reduction is performed after voice surgery. Your voice surgeon will likely encourage you to have the reduction first, but it is possible to do some reduction after voice surgery.

A Final Note

Patients should note that recontouring an Adam's apple is a very difficult, delicate procedure. Removing too much cartilage can permanently affect your voice. The good news is that this surgery generally yields an effective, satisfying, and permanent solution. In the hands of the right surgeon, this surgery can eliminate a common transgender issue.

12

Lower Jaw
(Mandibular) Surgery

A JUTTING OR RECEDING LOWER JAW can significantly diminish the aesthetic results of feminizing your face. If your lower jawbone *(mandible)* doesn't match your upper jaw and overall facial profile, the misalignment can detract from your overall look. Correcting your lower jaw length, by either surgically extending or shortening your mandibular bone, will improve an underbite or overbite, and will also improve your ability to chew.

Although a lower jaw's position has nothing to do with the skeletal differences between men and women, attending to it can improve your facial aesthetics considerably. Also, some patients with sleep apnea can benefit greatly from jaw surgery; the base of the tongue is attached to the jaw and moving the jaw forward increases the space for air to flow in the back of the throat. This can alleviate sleep apnea.

Lower Occlusion and Malocclusion

Mandibular or lower jaw surgery is usually employed to correct problems involving the length of the mandible and its relationship to the upper jaw *(maxilla)* and occlusion with the upper teeth. What is *occlusion*? It's how the surfaces of your upper and lower teeth come together at rest or during chewing.

When the alignment is correct, your upper teeth fit slightly over your lower teeth. Your lower teeth protect your tongue from being bitten when in normal configuration. Although correct occlusion results in a healthier mouth, very few of us have perfect occlusion. Most people, however, experience minor issues that don't need repair.

Malocclusion, on the other hand, is a much more serious misalignment of the teeth and jaws. Referred to as a "bad bite," it appears in at least two distinct ways. In *retrognathism* (an overbite), the upper jaw and teeth severely overlap the lower jaw and teeth because the lower jaw is abnormally short. *Prognathism* (an underbite) occurs when the lower jaw and teeth severely overlap the upper jaw and teeth because the lower jaw is abnormally long.

CLASS I MALOCCLUSION

CLASS II MALOCCLUSION

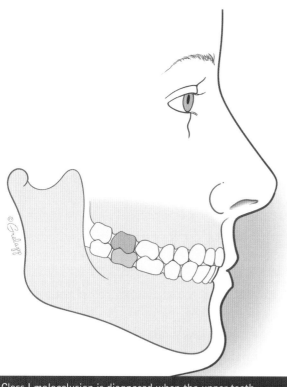

Class I malocclusion is diagnosed when the upper teeth slightly overlap the lower teeth.

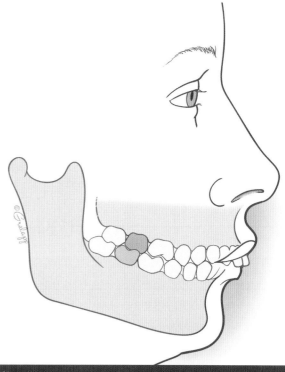

Class II malocclusion is diagnosed when a severe overbite is present.

In either case, malocclusion can cause a variety of problems, including speech and chewing difficulties and bite and breathing irregularities. These disorders can threaten the health of your teeth and gums as well as prompt pain and dysfunction in your *temporomandibular joint (TMJ)*. The TMJ joints connect the jawbone to the skull. Malocclusion can also leave you with an unfavorable appearance that detracts from the other changes you've made to your face.

You may often hear class designations in reference to occlusions and malocclusions. These designations further identify both the lower jaw length and position of the teeth, particularly the first molars. *Class I* refers to the desirable occlusion of the upper and lower jaws. In this case, the upper teeth slightly overlap the lower teeth

to produce what is considered a normal bite. More specifically, the *mesial-buccal cusps,* or first points of the upper first molar, fit nicely into the mesial-buccal grooves, or first indentations of the lower jaw first molar. The first molar in adults is the sixth permanent tooth on both sides of the upper and lower jaw.

Class II malocclusion refers to an overbite. In class II malocclusion, the lower first molar sits behind its normal position, creating both a receding lower jaw and chin along with a severe upper overbite.

Class III malocclusion is an underbite. In these cases, the lower first molar sits in front of its normal position, resulting in the underbite characteristic of an extended lower jaw that overlaps the upper jaw.

CLASS III MALOCCLUSION

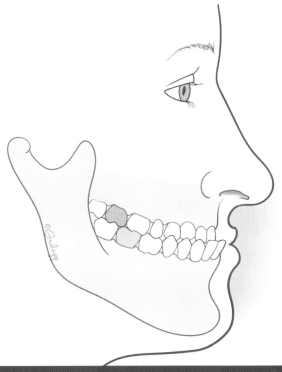

Class III malocclusion is a misalignment of the teeth in which the lower teeth are more prominent than the teeth in the upper jaw. This condition is also known as an *underbite*.

Abnormal jaw lengths can be caused by many factors—trauma, hormonal abnormalities, developmental issues, and even genetics. For instance, childhood or adolescent trauma to your lower jaw, and indirectly to your temporomandibular joint, may have caused a one-sided retardation or overgrowth of your mandible. Or a pituitary gland tumor may have triggered a growth-stimulating hormone abnormality resulting in an enlarged lower jaw. No matter the cause, there are surgical ways to correct either a jutting or receding lower jaw.

Other issues may also occur, including a very long face with vertical overgrowth of the upper jaw. Often, this is seen in combination with an overbite and is commonly described as *VME* or *vertical maxillary excess*. There are also several medical asymmetries of the jaw that cause the jaws to be tilted in one direction or another, while still maintaining a relatively normal dental relationship.

Undergoing Lower Mandibular Surgery

Most patients suffering from either a receding or protruding lower jaw undergo what's known as *orthognathic surgery*. Derived from the Greek word *orthos,* meaning straight, and *gnathos,* meaning jaws, orthognathic surgery is performed to straighten an improper jaw alignment and/or improve its function.

Although an orthodontist uses braces and other appliances to straighten crooked teeth, a surgeon uses bony osteotomies. Osteotomies refer to dividing a bone or excising a piece of bone to correct poorly positioned jawbones. Generally, both treatments are necessary. More

SURGICAL STEPS TO ADVANCE THE LOWER JAW

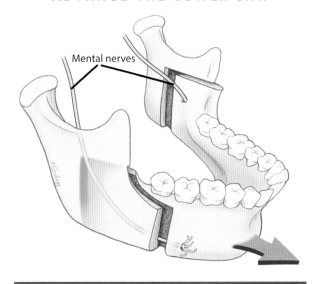

Mental nerves

Illustration shows where bone is removed to advance the lower jaw. Note the critical "mental nerve" that runs through the lower jaw and supplies nerves to the lower chin and lower lip.

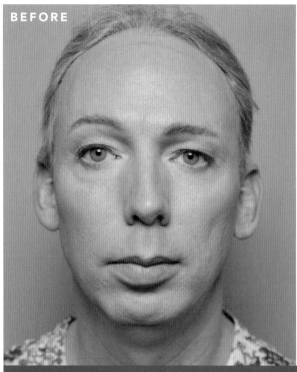

BEFORE

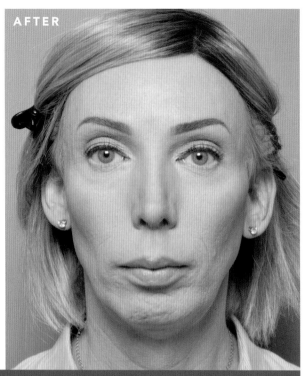

AFTER

This patient underwent facial feminization surgery for the upper face while being prepared for orthognathic surgery (bite correction surgery). Initial feminization procedures included forehead Type III contouring with scalp advancement and brow lift, feminizing rhinoplasty, upper lip lift, and thyroid cartilage reduction.

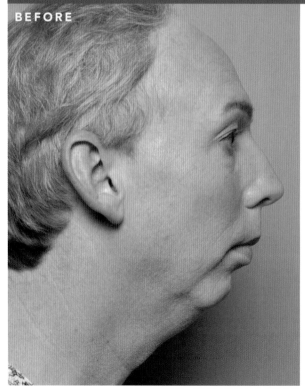

BEFORE

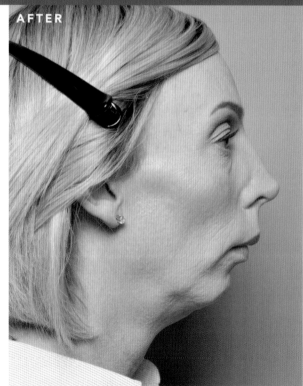

AFTER

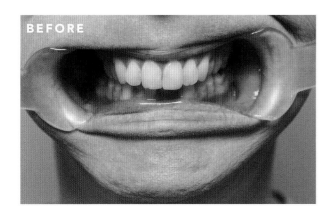

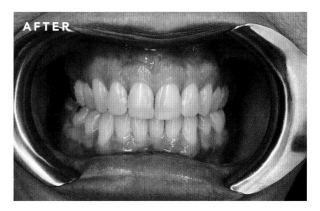

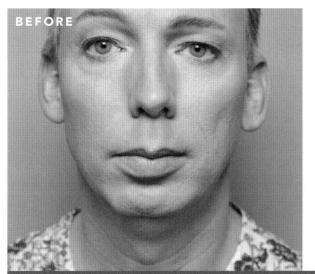

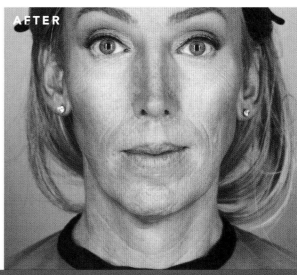

Same patient, shown on page 156, two years after bite correction surgery and a lower jaw advancement. The patient also underwent a chin reshaping.

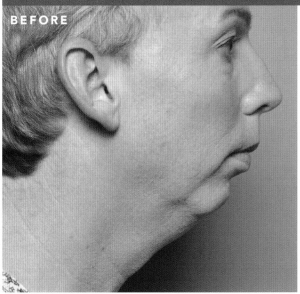

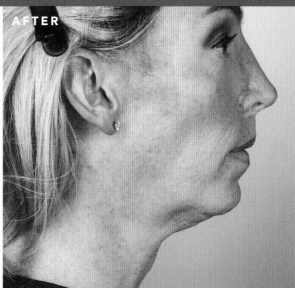

CLASS I OCCLUSION

BEFORE

AFTER

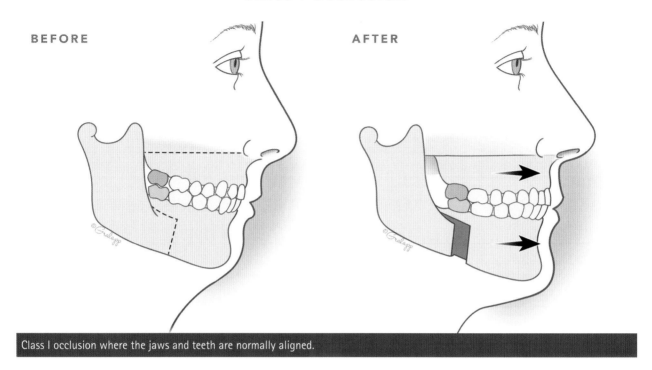

Class I occlusion where the jaws and teeth are normally aligned.

CLASS II MALOCCLUSION

BEFORE

AFTER

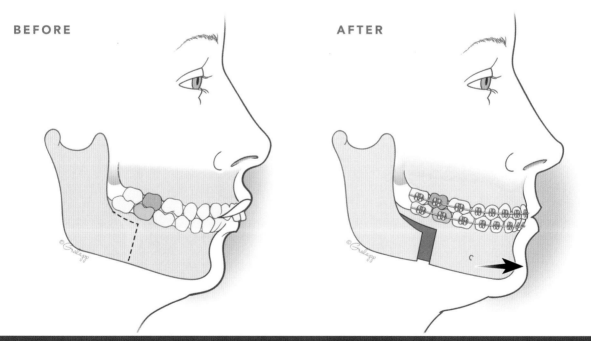

Class II malocclusion is diagnosed when a severe overbite is present.

PRE AND POST-OP CLASS III MALOCCLUSION

BEFORE

AFTER

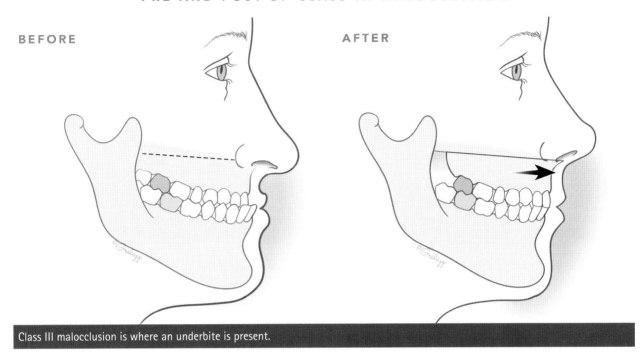

Class III malocclusion is where an underbite is present.

specifically, depending on your condition, your surgeon will recommend either a *sagittal split osteotomy* or a *vertical* (or *oblique*) *osteotomy*. Both these procedures involve entering through mouth incisions and cutting or splitting the lower jawbone. The jawbone is then moved forward if it is too short, or back if it is too long. By either lengthening or shortening the lower jawbone, your surgeon can improve its alignment with the upper jaw.

Although surgery is the primary treatment for lower jaw malocclusion, fixing an overbite or underbite also involves orthodontics. Sometimes, braces can correct the problem, but they are often not enough. Here's what you need to know about the entire process.

Collaboration Required

Mandibular surgery requires a multidisciplinary approach involving various health professionals: a dentist or pediatrician who usually diagnoses the problem initially; an orthodontist, who takes care of any pre- and postoperative teeth straightening; and then a craniofacial or maxillofacial surgeon, who performs the jaw-altering surgery. To measure the extent of the retrusion or protrusion, your surgeon will rely on cephalograms—detailed radiographic studies of the face—in planning your procedure. In addition, the doctor usually orders a set of plaster models of your teeth.

Orthodontics

Prior to surgically lengthening or shortening their jaws, most patients need orthodontics to reposition the teeth. Why? Because the surgeon needs to ensure that the teeth are situated in the upper and lower dental arches so that they fit together appropriately after surgery.

But does that mean every patient needs surgery after orthodontics? Not necessarily. Surgically repositioning your jaws as a follow-up to braces depends on the relative degree of your condition. It may be that a sliding genioplasty, the chin-altering operation we discussed in chapter 9, is enough to camouflage your overbite. Or a partial osteotomy—cutting and moving the jawbone to set back the front six teeth—is all that you need. In general, both orthodontics and surgery are necessary steps in correcting an overbite or underbite.

Mandibular Advancement for Overbite

To correct a receding jaw, the surgeon cuts or splits the jawbone at the back angle behind the teeth into two sagittal sections, the *medial* and *lateral* pieces. The medial piece lies closer to the midline or center of the face and contains the teeth. The lateral piece lies along the outside and contains the condylar or head of the mandible, which resides in the temporomandibular joint.

The medial or inner piece is then advanced forward to a new, more appropriate position while the lateral piece is left in place. The jawbone is then secured by inserting two to three titanium screws through the two bone segments at the angle. Many, maybe even most, surgeons rely on this method alone. In either case, the bone mends like a fracture with no external scarring, producing a beautiful profile.

Mandibular Setback for Underbite

A *sagittal split* can be used as effectively to set the jaw back as to move it forward. But we frequently use another technique, called the *vertical ramus osteotomy*. In this procedure, we cut the bone and move the jaw differently than we do with the sagittal split. We make an oblique cut through the ramus or vertical portion at the back angle and reposition the anterior or front bone segment backward.

We like the vertical osteotomy approach because it allows us to reposition the bone without causing major nerve injury. Such injury would lead to numbness in the lower teeth, lower lip, and chin. But we still choose the procedure based on the amount of setback we need to accomplish. In both the setback and advancement, the objective is to produce normal occlusion as well as an aesthetically pleasing profile.

When to Have Jaw Correction Surgery

If you are undergoing facial feminization, you would be wise to have your jaw correction surgery performed first. Then, you will need to allow at least three to six months for your lower face to heal before taking on other feminization surgeries. Moreover, these jaw correction procedures should not be confused with jaw tapering, angle reduction, or chin feminization—these procedures accomplish entirely different goals.

Repositioning the lower jaw either forward or backward is strictly for function and facial aesthetics, whereas recontouring the jaw and chin will enhance your look as a woman.

After Your Lower Jaw Surgery

As with any other face-changing operation, mandibular surgery should not be taken lightly. Whether your jaw is being set back or brought forward, the same postoperative steps are necessary to ensure a good outcome.

Recovery and Follow-up Care

Because these procedures are accomplished through the mouth, good dental hygiene is essential before and after your surgery to keep any infections at bay. Although you'll be given a prescription for antibiotics, brush your teeth at least three times a day to keep your mouth clean. We also tell our patients to rinse with an antibiotic mouthwash (Chlorhexidine) rather than alcohol-based mouthwashes.

Your stitches will dissolve on their own. Your incisions will leave no outside scars because the incisions are on the inside. Your bones should be solid again in six weeks. You may experience bruising and some swelling, but both will subside in about two weeks. It will be obvious from the initial swelling that you've had surgery, but that will soon be replaced by a better-looking lower jaw.

Diet/Activity

One of the most important postoperative instructions you'll hear after lower jaw surgery involves diet. Your jaws are usually not wired after surgery, but it is occasionally necessary. Therefore, you'll be restricted to soups and other soft foods for the next few weeks before graduating to solids. Patients should not be chewing during the early healing process, because it will disrupt what has been accomplished with the surgery.

You should also refrain from any physical strain for at least two weeks after the procedure. You should build up your physical activity slowly over the next month. Walking is very good for you. Other than these guidelines, expect some discomfort, although pain is relative. Our current pain management protocol will minimize your pain.

Side Effects and Potential Complications of Lower Jaw Surgery

Beyond the temporary swelling, bruising, and pain mentioned earlier, mandibular surgery is tolerated very well. Generally, there are no major complications, even though you may experience additional malocclusion and relapse, especially if your jaw is being advanced. Rest

assured that these incidents are rare. In fact, the issues discussed in this section are so unusual, that we haven't seen them in our many years of practice. However, be aware of the following possible problems.

Nonunions

Nonunion refers to a serious, and sometimes permanent, failure of a bone fracture or osteotomy to heal properly. It can occur when poor blood supply, infection, scar tissue, inadequate dietary intake, or excessive movement at the surgery site interrupts the normal healing process. Although a nonunion can arise with lower jaw surgery, it is very rare. If a nonunion surfaces, it likely will require corrective surgery.

Numbness of the Lower Lip

Numbness in the lower lip occurs when there is injury to the *inferior alveolar* or mandibular nerve. This is the nerve that supplies sensation to your teeth and, as it branches off as the mental nerve, supplies sensation to both your lower lip and chin. A sagittal split is designed to keep the nerve intact during the splitting process. Yet, when done incorrectly (and in some cases even if it is done carefully), the nerve can be injured. That injury, which can be permanent, can lead to numbness, particularly in the lower lip and chin area.

Anterior/Posterior Open Bites

An *anterior open bite* occurs when the front teeth do not touch each other, but the back teeth do. It is usually a result of the way that the jaw was fixed during surgery or healed. If the screws were placed inaccurately, they can cause a malocclusion that might require surgical correction or more orthodontics. A similar condition, called a *posterior open bite*, occurs when the upper and lower back teeth do not meet even though the front teeth are aligned properly. It is even rarer than an anterior open bite and may correct on its own without medical intervention.

Outcome of Lower Jawbone Surgery

Realigning the jaws and teeth produces aesthetically pleasing results, even if there may be small residual occlusion problems. Eliminating a prominent or receding lower jaw can have a tremendous psychological effect. Never have we heard our patients express even the slightest disappointment with their new profiles. However, this surgery does not eliminate the need for feminizing a masculine chin with a sliding genioplasty, should yours need modification. But mandibular or lower jaw surgery can give you a much prettier profile by correcting what nature gave you.

Commonly Asked Questions

I have had previous jaw surgery and am not happy with the outcome. Can I have it done again? Yes, you can have jaw surgery again. You might be at greater risk for complications such as nerve injury, but you can experience a successful outcome with follow-up surgery. Your surgeon, in collaboration with an orthodontist, may recommend preoperative orthodontics. Even if you've had braces before, preoperative orthodontics can improve the outcome in these cases.

My orthodontist has told me that I must have two years of preoperative orthodontics prior to surgery to correct my lower jaw alignment. Is there a way to shorten that time? Yes. Your orthodontics doesn't have to be completed before the orthognathic surgery. Sometimes, surgery may be undertaken with the understanding that the final bite may not be fully achieved. Also, the teeth will move somewhat faster after jaw surgery because the

metabolic potential of the bone is elevated for a period after surgery. After your jaw is surgically realigned, your orthodontist also has to bring your teeth into their final place.

I need my lower jaw set back and I also want facial feminization. I want to look as female as possible as soon as possible. Which surgery should be done first? We like to do the mandibular setback first, so the jaw is in its correct place before we start feminization surgery. We prefer this method, because the jaw position affects your profile.

I had orthodontics as a teenager, but it did not correct my underbite. Now that I want my lower jaw realigned, must I have braces again? Possibly. Sometimes, mandibular surgery works beautifully without additional orthodontics, a situation that is more likely when the surgeon is setting back the jaw, which is your problem. Sometimes, however, additional orthodontics are necessary. The choice depends on where the teeth are positioned at the time of your jaw surgery and how relevant the position of the teeth is to your jutting or receding lower jaw. Your surgeon will likely study your dental models and may refer you to an orthodontist for an opinion.

How long will it be before I see the entire results of my lower jaw surgery? After your surgeon brings the lower jaw into the right relationship with your upper jaw, you should see a pronounced difference in your profile immediately. You won't see the entire results, however, until your swelling fully subsides, which may take twelve to eighteen months.

I had orthodontics as a teenager and now, twenty years later, some of my teeth have gone back to their original position. I am not unhappy with my mouth. Would you be willing to see me for facial feminization surgery? Absolutely. It may be that we can work around your residual problems so that they will not be an issue.

A Final Note

Although malocclusions are no different in men than women, correcting these problems can have an enormous effect on your final facial aesthetics. A receding or overly extended lower jaw is simply not attractive, whatever your gender. Granted, in some people, the lower jaw looks abnormal only because the upper jaw (which we discuss in chapter 13) is set too far back or up too high. But when your lower jaw is causing the problem, a surgical correction is clearly needed to achieve an attractive face.

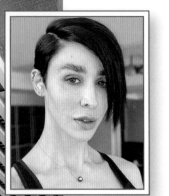

Autumn is a computer programmer and musician who underwent facial feminization surgery when she was twenty-nine.

WHAT PROCEDURES DID YOU HAVE DONE?

Scalp advancement, Type III forehead recontouring, feminizing rhinoplasty, sliding genioplasty, chin reduction, mandible contouring, surgical masseter muscle reduction, thyroid cartilage reduction, and fat transfer. I talked to Dr. Deschamps-Braly about doing hair transplants, and he urged me to wait until my FFS healed. So, I did that seven months after.

HOW DID YOU CHOOSE DR. DESCHAMPS-BRALY?

I consulted with a couple of local surgeons. One had done about five cases, and the other had done maybe fifty. One of the surgeons I met had a one-stop shop and did all trans surgeries. I felt that you can be really great at one thing or okay at a lot of things. I didn't feel super-comfortable with either of them, so I consulted with Dr. Deschamps-Braly.

I came across Dr. Ousterhout's work, and I was so impressed with how he understood the importance of the surgery. When I met Dr. Deschamps-Braly I thought he carried that as well. I could tell he wasn't just a surgeon. He had that meticulous nature about him, but he had an eye for aesthetics that was very similar to my own. The others I met were much more clinical. I also felt their approach was not aggressive enough. I was not looking for a subtle change. I was looking for dramatic changes.

I felt that Dr. Deschamps-Braly had the training, qualifications, the same aesthetic sense, and the right kind of demeanor and bedside manner. He really trusted me. I came in presenting male. He asked, "What's the plan?" And when I told him, he said, "Okay, great!" He wasn't ever trying to question whether or not I was ready for it. He trusted me, and that allowed me to trust him. I saw the number of cases he had done and his results, and I felt that he was the best I was going to find.

WHAT WAS THE PROCEDURE LIKE?

I was surprised how many people were in the OR running around doing things. That's when it hit me that this was going to be an event. Dr. Deschamps-Braly came in and we talked. He was genuinely interested in how I was feeling or if I had concerns. We were just kind of joking around as the sedative put me into a twilight sleep, and he had music on. I was very anxious, but it was very relaxed because he has such a good way of being. He was not distracted. He was very present with me.

The first thing I remember after, was his face about six inches from mine. He said, "It went great. I think you're going to be really happy. It went even better than I thought it would. Just hang in there and get through this." I'd had other surgeries, but I'd never had the surgeon be the first thing I saw. He held my hand, and it all felt really special. It takes a special kind of person to care about who's in front of them. That really stuck with me, even years later.

WHAT WAS RECOVERY LIKE?

Things got rough after that. I had drains, and I could barely swallow or talk. I was in a lot of pain after the first round of pain meds wore off, and I thought, "What did I just do?" That was a really tough period of time because I couldn't see any results yet. It was hard to be stuck waiting. I was released the next morning and things got much better right after that. In four or five days, the swelling started going down and I could see the initial results.

I'll never forget the day I got the bandages off. It was the most life-changing moment I've ever experienced. He unwrapped my bandages and took the cast off my nose, and said it was about as perfect as it gets. He handed me a mirror, and it was the first time I ever looked in a mirror and instinctively gendered myself female. I still looked a mess, but it was incredible. I don't think I appreciated how much dysphoria I had about the face I had to look at every day, and how uncomfortable I really was until I really saw myself as a woman for the first time. It was astounding, and I just burst into tears. Dr. Deschamps-Braly got pretty emotional, too, and I could tell he really cared to see how happy he made me.

I had lunch next door right after the bandages came off, and it was the first time I had ever presented as a woman in public. I'd say 85 percent of the swelling was already gone. I just looked like a woman who just had some work done. Over the next three to six months, the chin and jaw swelling went down and that part of my face became much more well defined. I had some swelling along the incision line at my scalp and that went down as things got better. By a month out, I was at about 95 percent of what I got out of the surgery.

I still have some numbness toward the front of my scalp, where it's just dull, but most sensation came back. Initially my lips and brow and chin were a little numb. My nose was a little stiff and didn't have a lot of feeling. But it's honestly nothing I ever think about. My jaw was pretty sore at first, but in a couple of weeks I was back to eating normally. I don't have problems breathing, but my nostrils are definitely smaller. My nose is definitely runnier than it was. It's nothing I ever notice unless I think about it.

WHAT ADVICE WOULD YOU GIVE TO OTHERS CONSIDERING THIS?

You can always make more money, and you can always pay back a debt. Money is something that comes and goes. Your face and your body and your life are not. A lot of people ask how I could afford it, or they think I'm rich or something. At the time I was making about $35 or $40 an hour. It was a complicated picture for me to put together. I sold my car and all my musical equipment, which felt like giving away my child. I got a second job. I got as many credit cards as I could, asked for credit increases, and maxed out all my cards. Most people aren't going to be independently wealthy or have extremely wealthy parents. That doesn't mean you can't do it. But you're going to have to figure it out.

A lot of Americans don't think about how little power you have to do anything if you go out of the country and something goes wrong. You have no legal recourse if something happens out of the country. A lot of people go and it's fine, but it's worth the money to go to the right doctor in the United States.

Don't try to micromanage your surgeon. Pick someone who's really good and has good vision and let them do their thing.

Don't look at this procedure like some sort of magic wand that's going to solve your depression, or issues with your father, and so on. It's going to help you present female better. That's it.

WHAT SURPRISED YOU ABOUT THE PROCESS?

It surprised me how quickly I was gendered female without making much effort. I'm six feet tall, so there are other things that facial feminization surgery can't change, but most daily interactions changed immediately.

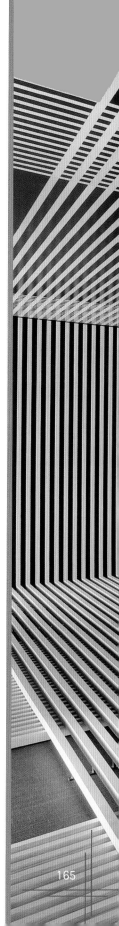

13

Upper Jaw (Maxillary) Surgery

YOU MAY NOT THINK THAT upper jaw *(maxillary)* surgery is a necessary step to transition from your birth gender to your new gender. Actually, there's nothing specific about your upper jaw that must be changed to help you appear more female. But like your lower jawbone, your upper jawbone can be malpositioned enough to affect your facial aesthetics; it can significantly diminish your new feminine look.

What can be done to bring your upper jaw in line with your other features, particularly your lower jaw? Fortunately, the upper jaw can be surgically moved in any direction, even widened and narrowed, to improve both the contact between your teeth and your appearance. Even if not medically necessary, this procedure may be a solution if you want to appear both feminine and attractive.

Differences in Male and Female Upper Jaw

The upper jaw or *maxilla* is generally no different anatomically in men than it is in women. Although it is larger in males versus females (just like other facial features), the contours and proportions are the same.

Why undergo surgery for the upper jaw? The maxilla and its associated *dental arch*, the curve shaped by the normal arrangement of your teeth, can be misaligned in several different directions. All these misalignments can affect your facial appearance and feminization results. Both the maxilla and its dental arch can be positioned too far backward or too far forward. They can be too far up or too far down. They can be asymmetrical to the right or left or rotated, meaning that the central incisors, your two front teeth, are located more to one side or the other. Finally, your maxilla and the arch can be too wide or too narrow. Misalignment of the upper jaw occurs for various reasons, the most common being heredity. Whatever the underlying problem, however, it can be corrected successfully with surgery.

Undergoing Upper Jaw (Maxillary) Surgery

Dentists frequently notice maxillary issues initially, but a craniofacial or jaw surgeon (trained as either an orthognathic or maxillofacial dental surgeon) will likely make the final diagnosis. To do so, your surgeon will use cephalograms to

CLASSIFICATION OF LEFORT OSTEOTOMIES OF THE UPPER JAW

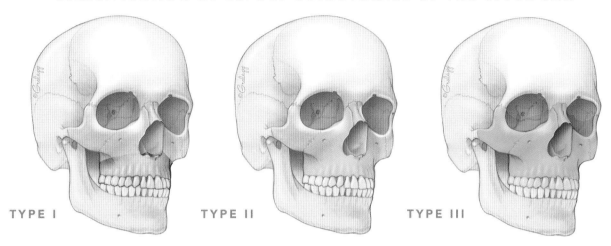

TYPE I   TYPE II   TYPE III

Classification of "LeFort" osteotomies of the upper jaw (maxilla).

evaluate both your bite and the aesthetic aspects of your jaw. With these studies, your surgeon will be able to confirm various issues associated with the maxilla, such as *short face syndrome,* a condition characterized by a shortening of the lower third of the face. This health condition is due in part to a deficiency or undergrowth in the upper jaw's vertical length. Like a man without his dentures, the upper teeth in these patients are generally hidden under the upper lip when the mouth is open.

Although most of our maxilla patients have short face syndrome, some individuals may exhibit the opposite condition, called *long face syndrome.* This condition is characterized by excessive show of gums and teeth when the mouth is open without smiling. The look is typically pronounced.

Whether your lower jaw is long or short, up or down, your surgeon can improve the placement and tooth show with maxillary surgery. Your doctor will consider many issues—bone, soft tissues, past procedures, and of course,

your preferences—in planning an operation that should improve your appearance.

A word of caution: Your problem may not be an upper jaw issue, but still may involve surgical repositioning of the lower jaw or both jaws. In any case, your surgeon needs to know your facial feminization plans because they will make a difference in your long-term, overall look. We have consulted with several patients whose original doctors were unaware that they wanted to feminize their faces.

These doctors made jaw recommendations based on cephalometric analyses of male measurements rather than female measurements. They did not understand, for instance, that setting the mandible back rather than moving the maxilla forward would lead to the best feminization result. Setting the mandible back gives the lower face the smaller proportions necessary after the nose is reduced and the forehead repositioned. In other words, advancing the upper jaw would be exactly the wrong strategy because it would enlarge the mid-face.

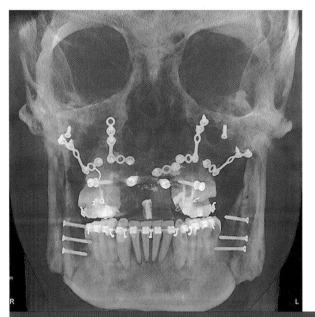
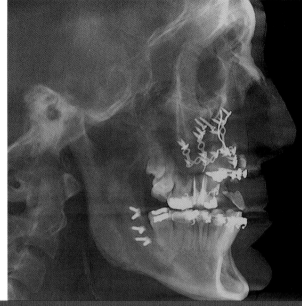

This patient had a class III malocclusion with a personal history of a cleft lip and palate that required a LeFort I (upper jaw surgery) and bilateral saggital split osteotomy (lower jaw surgery) for correction. These photos show the hardware required to secure the bones after the patient's bite was achieved.

SHORTENING OF THE UPPER JAW

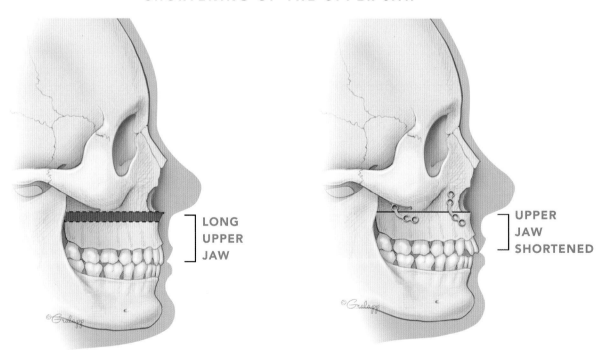

LONG UPPER JAW

UPPER JAW SHORTENED

Illustrations represent a patient with a vertically long upper jaw. The area in purple, on the left, shows where bone is removed. The illustration on the right shows how titanium plates and screws are used to the secure the bones.

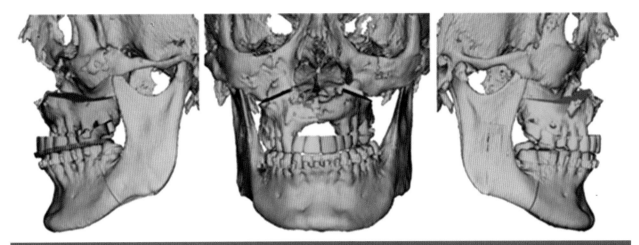

Surgical planning of complex facial bone surgery using rigid acrylic splints, which are prepared and printed on 3-D printers. Splints are used intraoperatively to position and provide a relationship between the upper and lower jaw to ensure the correct final position prior to internal fixation.

If you have any plans to feminize your face, but want to deal with your upper and lower jaws first, make sure you tell your surgeon. With the right planning and consultation, you'll achieve a result that will be in harmony with your new feminine look.

Orthodontics

Although the bony structural problems involving the upper jaw are not orthodontics problems per se, orthodontics is certainly part of the mix. No matter which maxillary malposition a person experiences, it can ruin the alignment of the teeth as well as detract from facial aesthetics. Because teeth straightening may be necessary with any upper jaw correction, it's extremely important for us to work closely with an orthodontist early in the process.

Unfortunately, many orthodontists think they can treat individuals with upper jaw issues with teeth straightening alone. But by overestimating their ability to correct a problem with appliances alone, they can make matters worse. How so? They fail to position the teeth properly on the

jaw's bony base. Or the teeth they move eventually fall back into place because the jawbone underneath was not surgically corrected. In either case, what often happens is that the orthodontist convinces the patients that they don't need jaw surgery (much to their relief!) when that is exactly what is required. By the time we see these individuals, they typically need more orthodontics as well as upper jaw-altering surgery.

If you have a maxilla problem, you will need a qualified jaw surgeon who can conduct a proper and thorough diagnosis and recommend possible treatments. By collaborating with an orthodontist who understands the dual role of maxillary surgery and orthodontics, and isn't hesitant to recommend both, this surgeon can produce an excellent result.

We prefer to work with orthodontists who are known to us; however, it is sometimes necessary to work with an orthodontist who is local to our patients. If you need jaw surgery on the way to your life as a different gender, the necessary preliminary orthodontic work can be coordinated with an orthodontist in the city

Having had previous FFS with another surgeon, this patient required multiple revision surgeries. Revisions included: Type III forehead contouring, brow lift, jaw contouring, jaw angle reduction, chin reshaping, and fat grafting.

BEFORE

AFTER

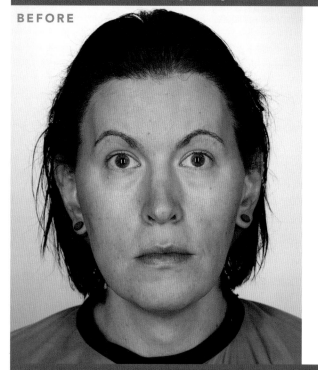

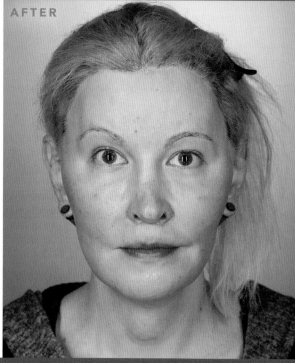

Revision surgeries, described above, adjusted the projection of the forehead, eliminating the appearance of deep-set eyes.

BEFORE

AFTER

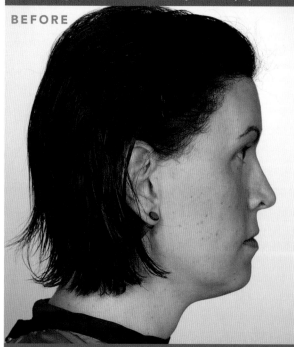

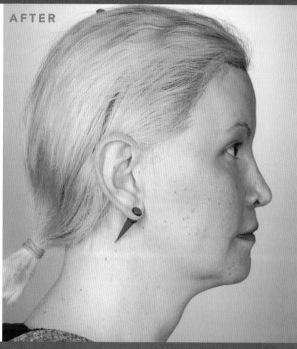

The Le Fort I procedure both shortened the lower segment of her face and gave her a "normal bite." The chin revision surgery was also required to shorten the vertical dimension of her chin.

where you live, although it may be significantly easier to have your orthodontics performed by someone who is familiar with the particulars of orthodontics in the context of a patient undergoing gender transition.

Surgery on the Dental Arch

No matter what the issue, the maxilla and its dental arch, the curve of the teeth, can be adjusted using one standard operation called a *LeFort I osteotomy*. Designed for reconstructing the mid-face, it relies on separating the teeth-bearing dental arch of the upper jaw from its bony attachments and repositioning it in a new location. The LeFort I osteotomy is an inpatient procedure accomplished with incisions through the mouth while the patient is under general anesthesia.

After entering the area, we make an initial cut across the entire upper jaw, just above the floor of the nasal cavity and the tips of the upper teeth. We then reposition the entire dental arch, which has been mobilized in one piece, in proper relationship to the lower jaw.

Depending on your needs, we may have to perform other steps. These steps may include removing further bone from the osteotomy site and/or grafting bone from the outer layer of the skull to fill any remaining upper jaw open space. Taking bone from the temporoparietal area of the skull also leaves a slight depression but that often fills over time. If not, the scalp hair hides any minor deformity.

In any case, the jawbone is then held in position by internal plates and screws, which remain for life. These plates and screws cannot be felt and are not magnetic, so they cause no problems if you go through airport security or undergo an MRI scan, for instance. They are no

different from the plates and screws we use in a sliding genioplasty. Unlike the lower jaw, wiring the dental arches together after this surgery is generally not necessary.

Unfortunately, not all issues related to the upper jaw can be corrected. The bone can be modified in some people with very long mid-faces, for instance, but there is no satisfactory way to reduce the excess skin without leaving a very noticeable scar from an excision across the mid-face. The good news is that when properly evaluated, most upper jaw issues can be addressed successfully. Like other facial procedures, this one must be performed with your other features in mind.

After Your Upper Jaw Maxillary Surgery

To ensure long-term success with an upper jaw surgery, you must take good care of yourself after the procedure. Many of the following cautions are no doubt familiar to you because they apply to every facial feminization procedure. Still, they bear repeating because your facial aesthetics and upper jaw function are at stake.

Recovery and Follow-up Care

Recovery from upper jaw surgery is similar to recovery from lower jaw surgery. Your stitches will dissolve on their own. You will not have any dressings, but you will have to take the antibiotics your surgeon prescribes. Remember to brush three times a day and rinse with antibiotic mouthwash (Chlorhexidine) to keep your mouth clean. (Do not use strong mouthwashes.) We control movement in these cases with elastics and rubber bands attached to the braces that your orthodontist applied, or we may use "arch bars" that conform to the arch of the teeth. As such, you'll have an easier time talking and eating, even though your diet for the next five or so weeks will consist of soup, eggs, mashed potatoes, and other soft foods.

The mantra for physical activity after this operation is the same as for any facial feminization operation. Take it easy for the next four weeks. If you have a desk job, you probably can go back in two weeks even though you'll be a little swollen. If you want to look perfect, wait another week or two.

Side Effects and Potential Complications of Upper Jaw Surgery

Maxillary surgery is typically a well-tolerated procedure that leaves patients with little to no pain, only moderate swelling, and bruising. Some people experience little or no discomfort whatsoever. Routine pain medications will manage any discomfort that may arise.

Although most individuals exhibit some discoloration for ten to twelve days, some people only have swelling. As with mandibular surgery, major complications with this procedure are very rare.

There are potential issues you need to keep in mind as you plan to undergo your operation. Among them, nonunion, a permanent failure of a bone fracture or osteotomy to fuse and heal properly, is probably the most significant problem you might encounter. Yet, none of our patients have experienced this complication. Nonunion after jaw surgery is extremely rare. As we described in chapter 12, a nonunion can occur after both lower and upper jaw surgery for the same reasons. These reasons include poor blood supply, infections, scar tissue, inadequate dietary intake, or excessive movement of the surgery site. Any of these issues can interrupt the normal healing process, eventually requiring additional upper jaw surgery.

Although major hemorrhaging is also a possibility with any maxillary surgery, it is exceedingly rare. Still, we prepare our patients for a potential transfusion, especially if they are having their upper jaws moved backward. This surgery is more likely to cause bleeding issues.

It is possible that post-surgery orthodontics may be necessary to make the final correction to your occlusion. This is especially true if you needed braces prior to your procedure. Your surgeon's recommendation will depend on how far the jaw is moved and in which direction. You may have an increased need for orthodontics if your jaw was moved forward, backward, right, left, or rotated, rather than upward or downward.

Outcome of Upper Jaw Surgery

The results of this surgery are both dramatic and uniformly pleasing. Although it takes ten to twelve days for the major swelling to subside, patients usually see a marked difference in their upper jaw immediately. Our transfeminine patients who have needed maxillary surgery have experienced a marked improvement afterward. Their facial proportions were enhanced. Their faces now appear narrower and a little longer than before surgery. These patients also sport an appropriate tooth show with better occlusion and a more acceptable profile.

Double Jaw Surgery

Double jaw surgery *(bimaxillary surgery)* is designed to reposition both jaws at the same time. This type of surgery is performed in about 50 percent of our orthognathic cases. There are certain situations where single jaw surgery alone is not appropriate. Essentially, the other jaw needs to be in an acceptable position for single jaw surgery to accomplish its mission. If there is a twist or vertical excess or a change

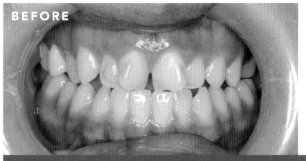
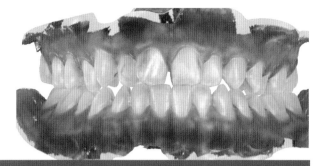

BEFORE

This patient had a LeFort I osteotomy with reconstruction and advancement during her facial feminization surgery. The photos demonstrate the orthodontic collaboration that is often required for this corrective surgery.

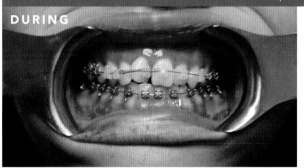
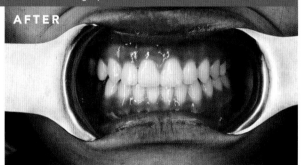

DURING

AFTER

in the occlusal plane is needed, then both jaws need to be operated on.

How do we position the jaws when both will be undergoing surgery? We start with one jaw and fabricate a custom "splint" to relate this jaw to the other one. After the first jaw surgery is performed in the operating room, the "splint" is removed and the second jaw is placed into position. A *splint* is a small wafer of acrylic material that has imprinted grooves that match your teeth.

We also use virtual surgical planning to complete a "mock" surgery on the patient, and our surgical guides are printed on 3-D printers. As a result, the time required for planning the surgery is reduced and the accuracy is significantly increased.

Commonly Asked Questions

I need to have my upper jaw repositioned, but also need facial feminization surgery. Which should I do first? In general, we like to do any corrective jaw surgery before facial feminization procedures, but we have done it in the other order. You'll need to allow several months for your face to heal before proceeding with any facial feminization.

How long will I be in the hospital following this surgery? We usually monitor our patients in the hospital for one or possibly two nights after their surgery.

Is there an age limit to this surgery? No, as long as you are healthy you should do fine with this procedure.

How do I choose the right surgeon? If you are a transfeminine patient, you need to make sure that the craniofacial surgeon you choose can perform this procedure expertly and understands the differences between the female and male face. The surgeon must be aware that you are transitioning and are undergoing facial feminization. No matter where you have your dental procedure, it's helpful to collaborate on the options with your selected surgeon.

Do I need to have my jaws wired together after this surgery? No. The plates and screws we insert usually are enough to stabilize the upper jaw. One plate is in the front on each side; one is in the back on each side. We also use elastics between the dental arches to prevent impaction.

When can I go back to work? You can resume a desk job within two weeks in most cases. If you are still a little swollen, wait another week. If you have a job that requires physical exertion, plan on returning in four to six weeks.

A Final Note

You do not need to reposition your upper jaw to look like a woman. You can feminize your face without undergoing major surgery on the maxilla, because the maxilla is anatomically the same in both genders. But will the changes that feminize your face be as effective if your upper jaw is out of alignment? The answer is no. Your entire facial appearance depends on every feature being proportional to each other. So, if you are planning facial feminization, you'd be smart to take care of the basics first.

14

Facelifts and Other Facial Procedures

YOU MAY BE INTERESTED, at some point, in other "standard" plastic surgeries to rejuvenate your face. Although procedures to lift your sagging eyelids, jowls, and other facial skin are not feminization techniques, they can significantly improve your facial aesthetics. The same is true of a surgery to pull back your protruding ears. It can totally change your profile. Additionally, because your teeth are an important part of your appearance, paying attention to them is key to transforming your face. Here's how these alterations can be the perfect finishing touch.

Facelifts

Known medically as a *rhytidectomy*, a facelift can help you appear healthier and younger than your years would suggest. But it is not a facial feminization procedure. It is not a substitute for reconfiguring the underlying bony structures of your face to make you appear more like a woman.

Some of our transfeminine patients have opted for facelifts in addition to FFS. This surgery entails sculpting and redistributing fat and muscles in the face, jowls, and neck, as well as in the deeper layers of the face. This can make the skin look tighter and younger. Along with a facelift, we also do work on the floor of the mouth—reducing the size of the *digastric muscles* (which run under the jaw), the deep fat known as *subplatysmal fat,* and the salivary glands under the jaw called *submandibular glands.* Together, these procedures provide improved results compared to older facelift techniques.

Facial Aging and Gender

Growing old may be a natural part of living, yet a phenotypic male face ages differently in some ways than a woman's face. Males tend to develop more fullness in the *submental area* or the area under the chin, creating excess skin and fat. Females generally develop more excess facial skin. What causes these changes is a very complex process, and there is still much unknown about it.

Scientists believe that gravity, genetics, and your overall health play a role in how your skin wrinkles and sags. Yo-yo dieting, smoking, sun exposure, lack of good skin care (specifically

FACELIFT AND NECK LIFT

BEFORE   AFTER

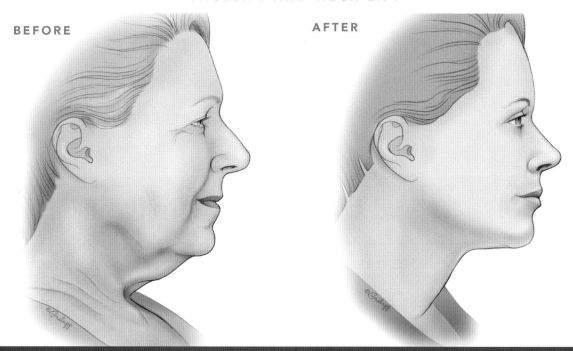

These illustrations show a patient who has had a facelift and neck lift. On the right, notice how the loose skin has been tightened.

SPF moisturizers), and even your attitude, affects your risk for wrinkles and sagging skin.

In time, all these factors may affect your skin's elasticity, firmness, and underlying bone, fat, and muscle support. We do not all age at the same time or in the same way, but eventually, we all begin to show sagging in the neck, jowls, and nasolabial folds—the grooves at the sides of the nose and the corners of the mouth.

How does aging affect a feminized face? It all depends on the facial area. The forehead is decreased in size during feminization, but the upper face does not show any aging afterward. The skin is actually tightened by the forehead procedure itself and/or an accompanying brow lift.

Your lower features, however, are a different story. As the lower jaw becomes smaller with feminization, it loses some tissue support.

Tightening this area cannot be accomplished during feminization. It takes at least three months after jaw tapering for the swelling and muscle mass changes to settle. If you are at an age when your skin still has sufficient elasticity, the excess skin left after that process will contract nicely.

Yet, if you are more mature in years (in your forties, fifties, or older), loss of elasticity will become an issue that might need attention. It can show up in early jowls, a fold of skin in your upper neck, or deeper nasolabial folds.

Timing of a Facelift

Whether or not you have undergone FFS, you may still wish to look younger. A facelift might be for you, especially if you are over forty. Still, if you are planning both surgeries, you shouldn't have a facelift sooner than six months after FFS. If you are trying to lose weight, the

NECK LIFT

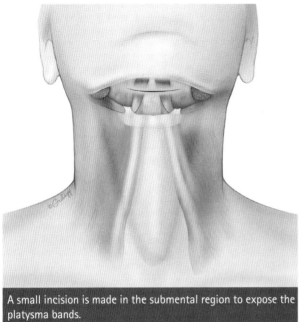

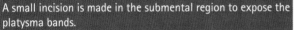

A small incision is made in the submental region to expose the platysma bands.

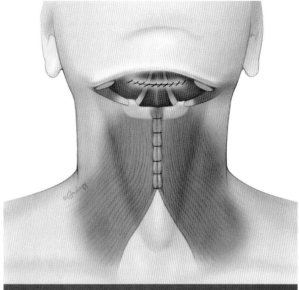

The platysma bands are sutured together to create a sling to support the structures and create a more youthful neck.

procedure shouldn't be completed until your weight is stabilized. If you lose weight after a facelift, some of it will come off your face. The loss probably will lead to excess sagging skin, and another facelift may be needed.

Undergoing a Facelift

There are many versions of the facelift, but the one most commonly used is known as the *SMAS,* an acronym for *superficial muscular aponeurotic system.* The SMAS is a deep, underlying layer of facial muscle and fibrous tissue. With this technique, the SMAS layer is lifted upward, separate from the skin, which is also pulled gently backward. The SMAS technique produces a very nice lift for jowls and redundant neck muscles. This procedure also tends to last longer than the traditional skin lift because it involves deeper layers.

This surgery can be performed under *twilight sedation* (conscious sedation that relieves

anxiety and reduces pain) with local anesthesia. Yet, our preference is to use general anesthesia, which provides the most patient comfort, particularly for surgeries on deeper layers of the face and neck. In addition, our patients stay in the hospital overnight, so they get excellent nursing care. The length of the operation depends on various factors, most notably what needs to be accomplished and how fast the surgeon can work. We usually complete an SMAS facelift in four to four and a half hours. We remove the facial dressings and drains the morning after surgery; sutures are removed on the fifth and eighth days.

Your surgeon will help you decide which procedure is best for you. You may not need a full SMAS, or you may benefit from other procedures, such as a *neck muscle plication* (a neck lift) with or without SMAS. Many creams and other treatments on the market today may help improve sagging and wrinkling skin somewhat,

COMMON FACELIFT PROCEDURES

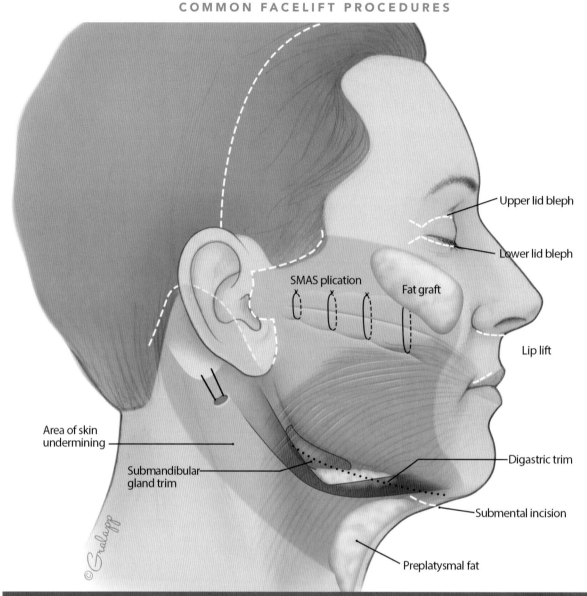

Upper lid bleph

Lower lid bleph

SMAS plication

Fat graft

Lip lift

Area of skin undermining

Submandibular gland trim

Digastric trim

Submental incision

Preplatysmal fat

Illustration shows some of the procedures associated with a facelift and the areas of the face commonly rejuvenated.

but they cannot produce the same long-term results as a facelift. Other therapies and procedures can also be performed.

Dermabrasion, an exfoliating technique to remove outer layers of skin, has improved skin quality and texture in our patients. Also, various types of chemical peels may be helpful. In addition, almost all patients benefit from the routine use of tretinoin, called *Retin A,* which is a derivative of vitamin A. It is the only skin cream currently sold that actually has a medically beneficial effect on the skin. It can reduce wrinkles and areas of darkened and rough skin that result from sun damage. Routine use of sunscreen is also part of any good skin-care regimen and may also protect the results of your surgery.

Fat Grafts: Improvements to Facelifts

Fat grafting has changed the way we do facelifts. Loss of volume in the face is a significant contributor to facial aging. The effectiveness of a facelift is multiplied by combining the tightening effects of skin removal along with the volumizing effects of fat replacement into the face. Fat grafts can be placed in areas such as the cheeks, the lips, the eyelid-cheek junctions, and the chin. Fat implants are also commonly used in the nasolabial folds.

One can think of the aging process as a combination of loss of skin quality, development of skin excess and volume deficiency, and descent (sagging) of facial tissue. All four issues need to be addressed in a facelift to obtain the best results. In neck procedures, it is also useful to debulk some of the muscles in the deeper portions of the neck underneath the chin to achieve the most aesthetic effects.

Side Effects and Potential Complications of Facelifts

Although a facelift is elective surgery, it is surgery just the same. You will have some degree of bruising and swelling. Your healing time will depend on your age and other factors such as how long it normally takes you to heal after receiving a cut or bruise. Count on a recovery time of two to four weeks before you can go out in public comfortably.

As with all facial surgery, you will be asked to sleep with your head elevated on two to three pillows for several weeks. Although you can shower and wash the incisions, you shouldn't wear cosmetics, other than moisturizers. Also,

be aware of the following complications that might occur after surgery.

Infection

Infections occur when patients fail to take their prescriptive antibiotics and/or are in poor health going into the surgery. To avert the problem, we insist that every patient take an antibiotic for a period after surgery. We will not operate on any patient who is not physically ready for surgery.

Hematoma

A *hematoma* is a blood clot that is often the result of a sudden increase in blood pressure during or after surgery. A hematoma can also occur when the blood pools or there is an issue with a drain placed near a surgery site. To avert a blood pressure spike during surgery, we tend to use a number of long-acting medications including clonidine, and anxiolytics to keep blood pressure in check. We also tell patients to restrict any straining activity (including sex) that might raise blood pressure in the weeks immediately following surgery.

To prevent any blood from pooling, drains are inserted during the operation. They are removed five days later at the first office appointment. Although drains may be removed sooner, we have found that patients have less swelling and bruising if they are left in a bit longer. We have each only had to take one facelift patient back into surgery in the past eleven years because the patient's blood pressure caused a hematoma. Three other patients had minor clots that were suctioned successfully in the hospital. All these patients did very well.

Facial Numbness and Paralysis

Temporary numbness, especially in front of the ears and along the hairline, can occur after

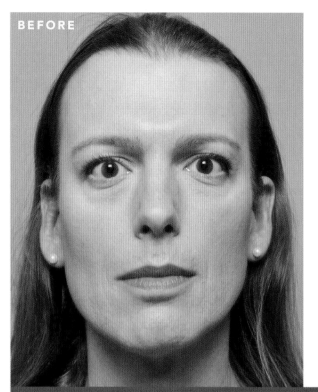

BEFORE

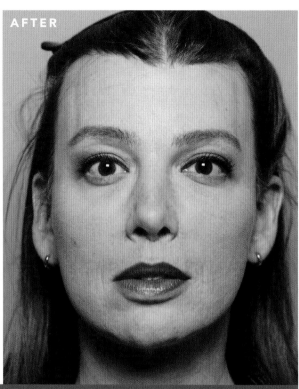

AFTER

The patient underwent a facelift following FFS surgery. FFS procedures included forehead type III contouring, scalp advancement, brow lift, fat grafting (fat injections) , rhinoplasty, upper lip lift (shortening) , chin and jawline feminization and thyroid cartilage (Adam's apple) reduction. Later she underwent a facelift, submandibular gland reduction and panfacial fat grafting (injections).

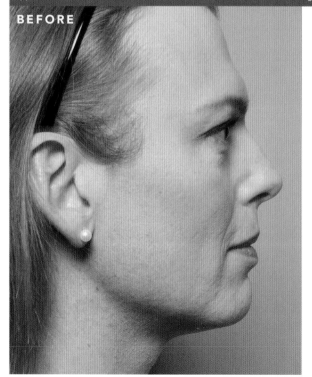

BEFORE

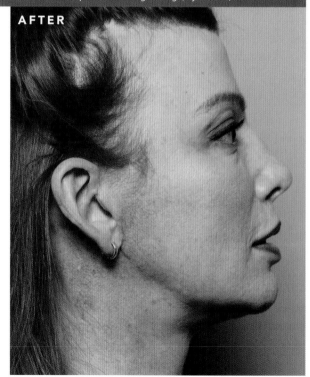

AFTER

facelifts because the sensory nerves under the skin are cut during the surgery. Eventually, sensation returns, even though it may take months, sometimes even up to a year. Facial paralysis, however, is a more serious issue. Facial paralysis is associated with facelifts that entail major tissue dissections and can result in a partial sagging of the face; this paralysis can be very frightening for patients, especially if they lose their ability to smile or wiggle their forehead.

However, the paralysis is usually temporary and usually lasts only for several months. Rarely, it is permanent. Facial paralysis is more likely to occur in a secondary SMAS.

Scarring

Scars are one of the most complex issues for any surgeon. How your body responds to an incision depends on how you heal and how well your surgeon performs the procedure. Does the surgeon put incisions in a conspicuous place? Are the sutures pulled too tight? What kind of material does your surgeon use? There's no question that some surgeons are better than others at making and closing incisions. Although a surgeon's technique does make a difference, a patient's healing is also a big factor.

For example, people with darker complexions are at higher risk for keloids and *hypertrophic scars* (thick raised scars) than people with paler skin. But those who have pale skin can end up with wider scars. Your surgeon should strive to give you the least conspicuous scar.

Skin Loss

Skin loss resulting from a facial cosmetic procedure is extremely rare. Yet, if a surgeon does not dissect enough skin, it can occur. Skin loss also can result from postsurgical infection, swelling, and either too much tension on the

incision or a restricted blood supply to the area. The latter is sometimes caused by smoking. Too much tension can also pull the earlobe down and result in an elongated earlobe. Still, with good surgical technique and follow-up attention, you should come through this procedure with flying colors.

Outcome of a Facelift

Although you will see changes immediately post-surgery, you may not realize your complete results for two to three months. One question patients always ask about facelifts is: "How long do they last?" In one sense, they last forever because the excess skin is gone for good. In another sense, however, they are only temporary since the aging process continues. Eventually, the jowls return, the wrinkles resurface, and the skin under the jaw droops again.

The reality is that nobody knows how long a specific facelift will "last." Obviously, the results in some people are more durable than in others. But in general, the same factors that aged your skin in the first place will govern how long your facelift lasts over time. We would hope most individuals would enjoy five to ten years of satisfaction with their appearance after a facelift. But there's a reality for people who live in year-round sunny climates, spending hours outside, perhaps without an effective SPF lotion. For them, the results of the first surgery may last only a few months.

A second facelift, however, may give them additional years of benefit. Why? The first procedure reduces the inherent elasticity in the skin to some degree, so it will take longer for the skin to sag again after the second procedure. No matter when and how often you undergo them, facelifts

For Facelifts and Nose Reshaping, Should I Choose an FFS Surgeon or a Plastic Surgeon?

To perform facial feminization surgery, your surgeon should first be board certified as a plastic surgeon. The surgeon who successfully performs complex FFS surgeries is highly trained and has expertise in both plastic and craniofacial surgery. With this experience, a FFS surgeon is probably a better choice for more routine facelifts and rhinoplasties than almost any other plastic surgeon. This observation is especially true for rhinoplasties. Even surgeons who specialize entirely in nose work seldom do a rhinoplasty that is as complex and demanding as those routinely performed during facial feminization.

are generally well-tolerated procedures that can add youthful years to your appearance.

Eyelid Lifts

Your surgeon may recommend an eyelid lift, known as a *blepharoplasty,* if your upper and lower eyelids are sagging and appear heavy. Although this popular cosmetic procedure often accompanies a facelift, it, too, is not a facial feminization technique. Still, it can add to your facial appearance by giving you a refreshed, younger look around your eyes.

Aging Eyes and Gender

There are differences between men and women as the eyes age. The differences are small but worth mentioning. Older people tend to have heavier eyelids, caused by drooping skin, fat, and muscle. As the brow descends with aging, particularly in males, it causes the upper eyelids to show excess skin. Sometimes this excess skin even obstructs vision. Older men frequently have a greater amount of protruding, bulging fat in their lower lids than older women. Whether you are a man or a woman, this look may give your face character, but the excess tissue is usually not attractive.

Timing of Eyelid Lifts

Before pursuing an upper blepharoplasty, you need to decide if you will first be undergoing forehead feminization surgery and a brow lift. If the answer is yes, you may not need to worry any further about your upper eyelids.

How so? When the brow is lifted, the upper lid excess skin will come along, causing it to virtually disappear. The contouring done to the bony upper outside angle of the eye socket during forehead feminization also markedly improves the appearance of the upper eyelids. Many transgender patients undergoing these procedures suddenly discover they no longer have excess upper eyelid tissue.

Yet, if you have an eyelid lift before your forehead is feminized, you will limit how much your surgeon can do in lifting your brows. The reason is that any excess skin has already been eliminated in the initial eyelid lift. If your surgeon tries to lift your brows farther, there's a real possibility that your eyes will not blink normally or close completely for sleeping.

An upper blepharoplasty may still be needed after your forehead feminization and brow lift, especially if you are an older patient. The amount of skin that needs to be reduced in a blepharoplasty will be markedly decreased, however.

The lower eyelids can be done either with FFS or at the time of a facelift. We prefer the latter, and usually combine it with another secondary

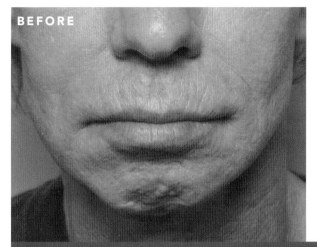

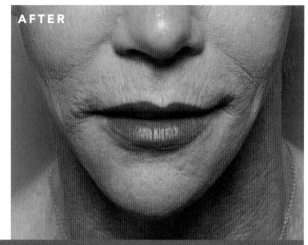

After previous FFS surgery a follow-up procedure was performed, including a face and neck lift, upper and lower eyelid lifts, submandibular gland reduction, and dermabrasion around the mouth. FFS procedures included scalp advancement, forehead Type III contouring, brow lift, rhinoplasty, jaw feminization, thyroid cartilage reduction, lip augmentation, upper lip lift, and pan facial fat grafting.

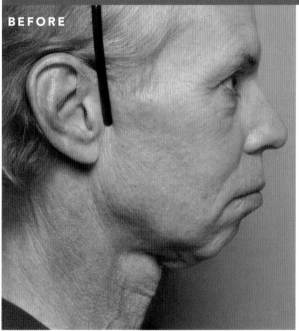

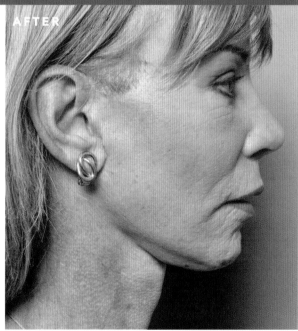

surgery such as further reduction of residual temporal baldness. This decision, however, is always based on your total feminization plan.

Unless there are special circumstances, we will wait at least six months after FFS to perform either a facelift or blepharoplasty. In older patients who don't want FFS, the procedure can be done anytime. Ideally, the surgeon and patient should collaborate on decisions about the type of surgery and its timing.

Undergoing Eyelid Surgery

Most older patients need the lower and the upper eyelids treated, but doing just one or the other can still produce a desirable result. During eyelid surgery, it is crucial for your surgeon to preserve and improve your normal eye contour.

With this procedure, the doctor removes or repositions any excess fat and skin. The doctor then reinforces the surrounding muscles and lateral canthal tendons that support the outer corner of the eyelid. A blepharoplasty can be completed under local or general anesthesia. If it is not accompanied by another surgery, it can be done very comfortably in an ambulatory setting without an overnight stay. If we do eyelid lifts in combination with other surgeries, patients must definitely stay overnight so a nursing team can care for them.

Recovery from Eyelid Surgery

Whether you are having work on your lower and/or upper eyelids, the postoperative care is the same. You need to elevate your head on two to three pillows until instructed otherwise by your surgeon. To reduce the swelling, we recommend applying four-by-four gauze compresses soaked in ice water to the eyelids. These compresses not only keep the lids clean, but also absorb the minor blood oozing immediately after surgery.

On the day following surgery, we have our patients start squinting and doing massage exercises in the eye area. These controlled movements help reduce the swelling following surgery and get the eyelid muscles functioning again. The sutures are removed on the fourth day. Bruising is usually not severe. Although you will have swelling afterward, you should be able to go out in public within eight to ten days.

Side Effects and Potential Complications of Eyelid Surgery

Complications related to a blepharoplasty are rare when the surgeon has the appropriate experience. But you still should be aware of at least some of the possibilities. *Ectropion,* or pulling away of the lower eyelid from the eyeball, can occur. This condition usually responds to nonsurgical management even though it may, on occasion, require corrective surgery.

A lower eyelid retraction occurs when the portion of the lid on the outside of the pupil is pulled downward. As a result, a greater portion of the sclera, or white of the eyeball, can be exposed. This complication can be difficult to manage and may require surgery.

To avoid both these complications, your surgeon should use a conservative approach for excising tissue around the eyelid. We would much rather tell a patient that we need to go back and take out more skin than tell a patient that we need to go back and correct the surgery with a skin graft.

Blindness linked to this surgery is extremely rare. One of the reasons we like to monitor our patients in the hospital right after their blepharoplasty is that we can check for any excessive bleeding. If not addressed immediately, bleeding can put pressure on the optic nerve, causing damage and even loss of sight. None of our patients has ever suffered significant vision loss or any other serious complication from this procedure.

Outcome of Eyelid Lift

Blepharoplasties are well-tolerated surgeries that can produce beautiful outcomes. As with every cosmetic procedure, however, you, the patient, must choose your surgeon wisely. If you do, you are very likely to obtain excellent results.

Otoplasty to Correct Protruding Ears

If you are put off by the way your ears protrude, you needn't be any longer. With a standard

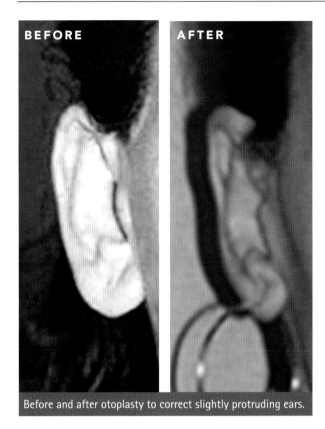

BEFORE | **AFTER**

Before and after otoplasty to correct slightly protruding ears.

surgery called an *otoplasty*, your surgeon can reduce the prominence of the pinna, the outside cartilage and skin structure that funnels sound to the middle ear. The end result is often that ears lie flatter, closer to the head.

Ear Size and Gender

Prominent ears have no relation to gender. Neither women nor men have a monopoly on this problem. Prominent ears usually occur when the *conchal cavity*, the seashell-shaped outermost part of the ear, is too deep. As a result, the ears protrude too far from the skull.

Other landmarks, such as exceptionally long earlobes and/or a flat *antihelical rim*, the ridge directly inside the outer rim, can also distort the ear. Yet, the most common complaint we hear from most adult transgender otoplasty patients

is that their ears stick out too far. A little protrusion is nothing to worry about for some people, but even the smallest prominence can be a big issue for others. Women tend to have an easier time disguising their ears because they can always cover them with longer hair. But if you look better in a short hairstyle, your ears can detract from your attractiveness.

In fact, many adults with beautifully sized and shaped ears once had the same prominent ears and profile that you may have. They most likely had their oversize ears pinned back as children.

Undergoing Ear Reduction Surgery

Otoplasty, the cosmetic procedure your surgeon will recommend to change the appearance of your ears, can take many forms. Surgery may involve cutting away tissue between the ear cartilage and skull to pin your ears closer to your head. Or, it may require reshaping the cartilage inside the "bowl" of the ear to create a normal antihelical rim. Ear reduction surgery may even entail reducing the length of the earlobes. Although this chapter does not discuss each procedure in detail, you should know that a competent plastic surgeon can successfully correct these issues.

In most otoplasties, the surgeon starts by cutting in the skin crease between the back of the ear and the head. From there, the surgeon can score and/or remove the necessary cartilage to reduce the ears or pin them closer to the skull. The back-of-the ear incision is often the only one your surgeon makes. Other cuts, such as on the lobule, may be necessary—depending on your ear issues.

Most of these surgeries are performed in an outpatient setting, but some may require hospitalization, especially if you are combining other procedures. Similarly, the type of anesthesia your surgeon recommends will depend, in part, on the problem being treated. Choices include local anesthesia, local anesthesia combined with intravenous sedation, and general anesthesia.

Recovery from Ear Reduction Surgery

The incision is closed with sutures that dissolve on their own. The ears are then wrapped in a bandage that must stay in place for four to five days. After it is removed, you can shower and wash behind your ears. For the next several weeks, we ask our patients to wear a headband (like a ski headband) at night to keep the ears immobile. After surgery, patients take a prescription antibiotic and pain medication to relieve the throbbing they are likely to experience for the first few days. Most patients respond very well to these surgeries.

Side Effects and Potential Complications of Ear Surgery

Although swelling and bruising occur with an otoplasty, both are minimal and usually disappear within eight to twelve days. Some individuals may experience numbness for a brief time. Although infections can occur, our patients have not experienced any infections. The normal scars are usually well hidden behind the ear. If the scars are in front of the ear, they usually become less obvious over time. Secondary revisions are sometimes necessary, but unusual. There are usually no complications.

Outcome of Ear Reduction Surgery

Over the years, we have treated many patients, especially children, with prominent ears. We have corrected the outward flaring in transfeminine individuals, with uniformly satisfying results. None required follow-up surgery.

Although absolute symmetry with these surgeries is impossible, we have managed to align the ears so that only someone with a ruler would see any discrepancies. In many cases, we've reduced earlobes in combination with a facelift. Even in combination, these procedures have yielded good results with few complications.

Cosmetic Dentistry

Throughout these chapters, we have focused on changing and improving all aspects of your face. But we must also comment on another feature that can significantly affect your appearance: your teeth.

Having great teeth is not necessary in facial feminization. But, as with the other surgeries we just discussed, a beautiful smile can round out your new look. Teeth that are nicely aligned and properly sized and shaped for a feminine mouth, will add to your new appearance. That's not to say you need the brightest white teeth in town. In fact, as people age, their teeth naturally become shorter, darker, and increasingly yellow. So, having the glistening pearly whites of a fifteen-year-old when you are fifty, is not realistic. Instead, aim for a smile that's clean, bright, and appropriately white for your skin tones and age. Similarly, crooked, chipped, or even missing teeth can make you look unkempt.

There are small differences in teeth when you compare men and women. In simple terms, females have narrower teeth than males due to their smaller facial bony structures. Their teeth must fit their jaw configurations.

Clean, white teeth and healthy gums go a long way toward improving your smile. Properly brushing at least two and preferably three or four times a day should be on your priority list. You should also floss regularly.

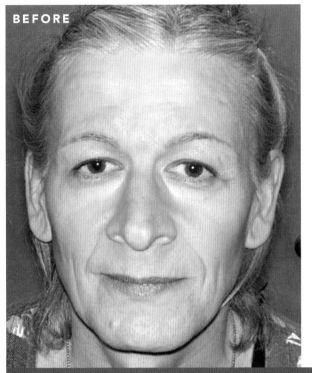
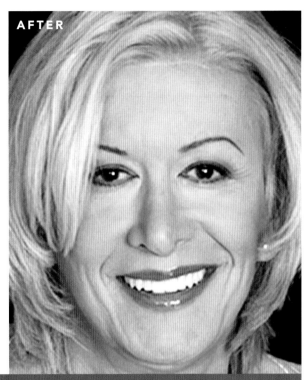

On left, before cosmetic dentistry and FFS procedures. On right, after cosmetic dentistry and FFS procedures: facelift, eyelid lifts, scalp advancement, Type III forehead contouring, chin feminization, nose reshaping, upper lip reduction, jaw tapering, and thyroid cartilage reduction.

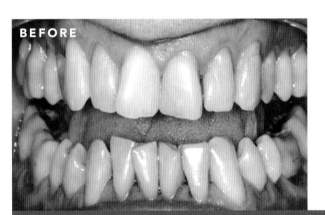
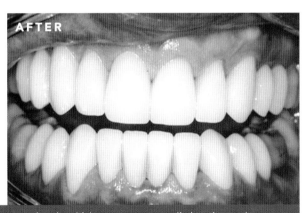

On left, the same patient prior to dental work. On right, after dental restoration, in which veneers were applied to the teeth. Cosmetic dentistry was completed by Dr. Samir Ayoub, San Francisco, California.

Make sure you visit your dentist regularly—at least once or twice a year—and more if your diet includes coffee, tea, and other foods that stain enamel. Besides making sure that your teeth are professionally cleaned, your dentist will check to see that your gums and supporting structures are free of infection and are healthy. The puffy, red, bleeding gums of gingivitis or periodontal disease are unsightly, will give you bad breath, and may even lead to rapid tooth loss.

Your dentist can advise you about other ways to improve your smile. Sometimes, simple contouring or shaping rough edges and crooked teeth can have a dramatic result at nominal cost. Other procedures include the following list.

Cosmetic bleaching, lightening, or whitening your teeth. Today's treatment options are many and varied, so there should be one out there that matches your lifestyle and budget. If you are willing to work with your dentist, a brighter smile can be yours.

Orthodontics. Braces can help your smile tremendously by aligning your teeth and giving you a beautiful bite. Unlike years ago, when only teens sported "tin grins" or "metal mouths," today there is no age limit on mending a crooked smile. *The caveat:* Straightening teeth takes time (sometimes more than a year), so you may wish to consider another method—laminates and veneers. They can yield considerable improvement in your alignment without the time needed to move your teeth. With today's veneers, laminates, and caps, your dentist can markedly improve the alignment, shape, length, and whiteness of your teeth. Crowns and bridges can be used to replace broken, poorly restored, and missing teeth.

Full mouth reconstruction—rebuilding and replacing all the teeth—can be expensive, but you still can get marked improvement without making a large investment. In addition, your surgeon and dentist can coordinate a program that helps you achieve the proper "tooth show" for a woman.

Remember, even if your teeth are worn down with age, they don't have to look undersize or unsightly. With proper oral hygiene and the right cosmetic improvements, you can have a winning smile that does justice to your new face.

Commonly Asked Questions

I want a facelift now, but I may do my FFS later. If I do it in this order, will I need another facelift? If you undergo jaw tapering, reducing the bony structure and support in your lower face will cause excess skin to accumulate in the upper neck area. That may mean another facelift could be needed. We recommend you do the FFS first.

If I have had a Botox injection, how long should I wait before having a facelift? Wait at least three to six months for the substance to clear your system, even though you may have a different experience as to how long it lasts.

Why is it important to plan an eyelid lift around other forehead feminization surgery? You'll want to think about your schedule, because skin needs to be excised with both procedures. If you do the eyelids first, your surgeon may not be able to do much with the brows.

When can I get my ears pierced after an otoplasty? Any time you are having surgery, it is unwise to undergo a procedure that might lead to an infection. Our advice to patients is that they shouldn't have their ears pierced for one to three months after their otoplasty.

Can an otoplasty be performed with other FFS procedures? Yes, we frequently combine it with other procedures, and this approach has never been a problem for our patients.

I have keloids in my earlobes from previous piercing. Can they be treated? Keloids, which are markedly overgrown scars, are difficult to treat, even though surgeons have tried various methods. None of the current treatments, such as steroid injections, radiation, or surgery, are uniformly successful in repairing this type of tissue overgrowth.

A Final Note

We have said often in this book that our goal is to give you the best aesthetic look possible. Obviously, every surgery that we have discussed, including the cosmetic procedures addressed in this chapter, are elective. Which procedures you decide to do will depend on your priorities and what you can afford. But as surgeons who have helped hundreds of trans-feminine patients, we can tell you that lifting your face and eyes, reshaping your ears, and/or achieving a clean, bright smile, can have an enormous impact. We know these can be costly and time-consuming procedures. Yet, they can also be the perfect finishing touch for your new facial features.

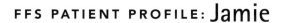

Jamie is a radiologist who had facial feminization surgery when she was thirty-seven years old.

WHAT PROCEDURES DID YOU HAVE DONE?

I consistently presented female more or less starting around the time of the surgery. I had started hormones, intermittently, about ten years before surgery though, I had been on full-dose hormones for less than two years. I started coming out to friends and family about a year before the surgery, but I didn't come out at work until after. I think I waited until then because when I looked in the mirror, I didn't see my reflection as female until after the surgery.

I had forehead contouring, and as part of that, Dr. Deschamps-Braly also did the contour of the upper nose to match because he took a centimeter off the brow forward projection. At the scalp incision he moved my hairline forward a couple centimeters. Then a lip lift and jaw reduction—about a centimeter off the bottom of my jaw.

HOW DID YOU RESEARCH THIS?

I'm a physician, a radiologist, so I do a lot with medical imaging. I read a lot about the science of it, and I had multiple consultations. I had one in Boston, and then I had another from a group in Spain. The other consultations had emphasized, "Oh, you're going to be so beautiful after this," and sort of hyping up their outcomes.

Dr. Deschamps-Braly was my third consultation. He said, "This is the science of how instant recognition of gender works. These are your measurements, and these are the things I think I should tweak. This is why I think it will work well for you." And yes, he also said, "I think you will be beautiful." But it was almost a side issue and more about, "This is how I will feminize your face. These are the practical considerations." There's a reason he's doing each component of the surgery, and as a whole it made sense to me. He was so meticulous and so numbers-driven, and also at the same time so warm and personable. I concluded that day there was no question; I'm going to go with him.

WHAT OTHER FACTORS IN THE CONSULTATION INFLUENCED YOUR DECISION?

When he started discussing the pros and cons of the various components of my potential surgery, it gave me insight into how he operated. He peeled back the curtain about what he was thinking, which was fundamentally about why he does what he does. That appealed to me as someone who researched facial feminization from the same approach to figure out what I wanted for myself.

HOW WOULD YOU DESCRIBE THE PROCEDURE AND THE RECOVERY?

I don't have any memories of the first twenty-four hours because of the sedatives and anesthesia. I was glad to have people I knew with me. I had clear instructions on what I was doing. The postoperative plan was communicated and planned out well, from what diet I was going to be eating, the supplies I got sent home with, the schedule for follow-up—it was all very well organized.

It's one thing to talk about what to expect after surgery, and another thing to live it. The initial amount of numbness really felt like a lot. Sensation has come back since then, but the experience of numbness was strange, especially in my forehead and my jaw. I was drooling a lot because of the decreased control over my lips and because there's not enough sensory input! The lips themselves were okay, but everything around the lips was numb—very strange, like it was a foreign object.

Now it's all basically back to normal. For a couple of months after, I would tap my chin to see if the sensation was returning, and after about four weeks I started to feel tingling. I thought that was a good sign; the nerves were working, even if they were not giving a complete signal yet. It took about six months to go from patchy numbness to sensation, and about eighteen months until I did not even notice any change from baseline sensation.

My forehead was numb in front of the incision for a while, but that completely returned. My scalp now has some sensation from the crown to behind the hairline incision, but it has not fully returned to baseline. Everything else feels the same. I've thought about getting some hair transplants to hide the incision, but it hasn't bothered me much to this point.

HOW HAS THIS SURGERY CHANGED YOUR LIFE?

I don't think I could have transitioned without this. It was so incredibly essential for me to reverse some of the effects of testosterone to really see myself. It enabled me to transition in a way that I truly had not envisioned was possible. It's hard to overstate the extent to which people's unconscious perception of gender affects how they interact with someone. There was no way I was going to get implicitly gendered correctly without this surgery. I'm over six-and-a-half feet tall. I felt I needed a face fully within the range of feminine facial measurements, particularly in the key aspects of facial feminization: the way light falls on the eyes and cheek because of the shouldering of the orbital ridge, the shape of the mandible, the length of the upper lip, and the size of the overall face. I think all of those key aspects have substantial basis in testosterone-mediated male/female dimorphism. I wanted to be solidly in the female ranges of those proportions as a starting point to get appropriately gendered social mirroring from other people.

WHAT ADVICE DO YOU HAVE FOR OTHERS CONSIDERING THESE PROCEDURES?

Everyone's experience is so different, from different ages to different situations. It's hard to know. I was in denial and upheaval for decades before I finally took the plunge. Even though I knew who my actual self was since I was a teenager, it wasn't until age thirty-seven that I came out. If you are young enough when you transition maybe you won't have much testosterone-related bone deposition of your mandible and orbital ridge. If it was a decade or more, it's very likely your bone structure is one of the main issues.

Don't restrict yourself from getting information. That includes talking to the people who are doing it and also other folks considering it. Don't be afraid of it.

The media plays up this trope of the "artificiality" of surgery, so many of us want to wait until they have the "full effect" of estrogen. Surgery is not artificial. It's reconstructive. It's mostly reversing the osseous effects of a hormone we never chose. As a radiologist, I see postoperative imaging from various surgeries all the time. People are getting things taken apart and put back together and reconstructed all the time. I'm not saying this is a minor thing. But it's great that medical progress has enabled control over how our bodies work and look and how they affect our lives.

When we get implicit recognition of our gender, we get the social cues that help us open our authentic selves to the world. I'm hoping for the day when there is less "othering" of people who are visibly trans, but we have a long way to go in the broader cis-centric culture. For some of us, the confidence and strength we gain will lead us to more visibility—paradoxically when we are less visibly trans in appearance. But we ourselves are the only ones who know our own point of view and our own needs, so we are the best judges of what we require from our gender presentation. When our physical appearance is in congruence with our internal self-image—which indeed can change over time—we can bring our best selves to life.

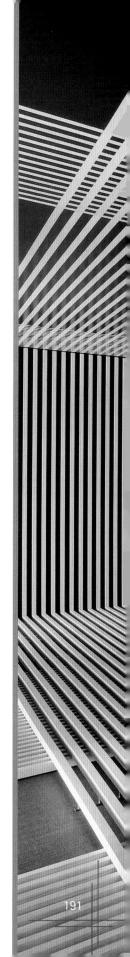

15

Hair Transplants

BY SARA WASSERBAUER, M.D.

WHY IS A FEMALE HAIRLINE important? Because nothing feminizes a face more subtly than the hairline. If you think of a face as a work of art, the hairline is the "frame." Reshaping a hairline, or adding to it in the case of hair loss, is a cornerstone of a completely feminine facial appearance. When patients decide to transition to life as a woman, the question of what to do with their hair, is one of the primary issues discussed.

Planning for Hair Transplants

As with all phases of facial feminization surgery, planning the procedures is important. There are several factors to consider with hair transplantation.

- *Female hairlines are lower than male hairlines and have a characteristic shape that subtly influences the perception of a face as female.*

- *Hairline feminization can be accomplished through a combination of surgical and nonsurgical techniques.*

- *Transgender patients need a plan for developing and maintaining their hair characteristics. Hair and hairlines change over the years, so a long-term plan is best and it's part of a comprehensive approach to the transgender transformation.*

Characteristics of a Female Hairline

A female hairline differs from that of a male hairline in several ways. On average, the female hairline is 5.8 cm above the center point of the eyebrows, although this can be higher, up to 7.8 cm. A male hairline typically is 7.1 to 9.9 cm above the center of the eyebrows.

Widow's Peak

Another defining feature of a female hairline is that 81 percent of the time it is shaped like a little "V" in the middle. This "V" is the *widow's peak*—named for the superstitious belief that having one was an early predictor of widowhood. The term "widow's peak" also might have referred to a mourning cap that was worn by widows dating back to the 16th century.

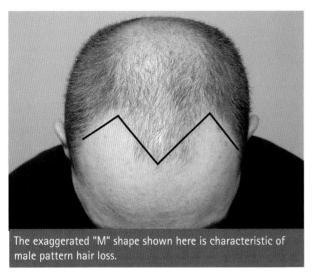

The exaggerated "M" shape shown here is characteristic of male pattern hair loss.

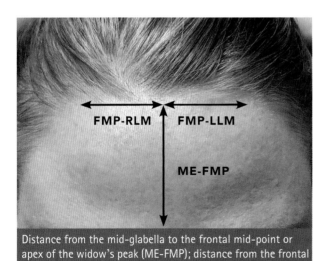

The temporal peak of a common female hairline showing fine and wispy hair that is characteristic of this area.

Male pattern hair loss has characteristic recession in the temples area, creating an artificial shape that mimics a widow's peak. Another way to describe this is as an exaggerated "M" shape. The areas of recession at the temples—the top points of the "M"—are called "temporal triangles," or "temporal peaks."

Temporal Peaks

Temporal peaks are full of fine and often wispy hair in female hairlines. They are characterized

by waves—known as *cowlicks*—and have several common shapes. The most common shapes by far are concave triangular (61 percent) and concave oval (26 percent). Hair in the temporal peaks of female hairlines is also less dense, providing the frame of the female face with a soft halo effect.

You can often faintly see scalp through the hair in this area. This is good news for those patients transitioning from male to female who also have some pattern hair loss. The goal of a feminized hairline is easier to accomplish when the characteristics of the male recessed hairline can be integrated into the final result.

Lateral Mound

Between the temporal peaks and the widow's peak, female hairlines also have a tiny mound of hair called the *lateral mound*. They are diminutive to be sure, about 2 cm wide and 1 cm high, so they typically go unnoticed. Most of the time these little mounds exist in pairs—like dimples on each side of a smile—but they can occur alone (and when they do it is usually on the right side). Whether they are flying

Distance from the mid-glabella to the frontal mid-point or apex of the widow's peak (ME-FMP); distance from the frontal midpoint to the apex of the lateral mound on the right (FMP-RLM) and on the left (FMP-LLM).

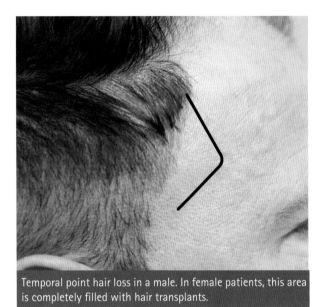

Temporal point hair loss in a male. In female patients, this area is completely filled with hair transplants.

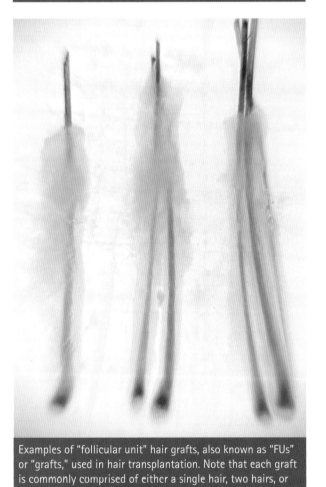

Examples of "follicular unit" hair grafts, also known as "FUs" or "grafts," used in hair transplantation. Note that each graft is commonly comprised of either a single hair, two hairs, or three hairs.

solo or have a wingman, lateral mounds are key, because they occur in female hairlines a whopping 98 percent of the time.

Temporal Points

Even more frequent in female hairlines than the lateral mounds are the *temporal points*. These are the strong arrow-shaped points of hair that seem to direct a profile observer straight to the eyes of the subject. When left to grow long, this is the hair that becomes "tendrils" in front of the ears. According to one detailed study of female hairlines, they are present in 100 percent of subjects. For transgender women, the temporal points present a problem. The reason is that the early stages of male pattern hair loss will significantly thin or sometimes even eliminate the hair in this area.

Another problem within this area is the presence of beard hair. The texture of beard hair is typically coarse and wiry, and often extends up from the jaw to meet the hair in front of the ears (sideburns as an example). It often cannot be used to mimic female hair in this area due to its texture and caliber.

Patients will typically choose to remove this hair with a laser or electrolysis. However, elimination of the beard and sideburn hair leaves a patient with the opposite problem. Male-to-female patients who have all their beard hair removed, need to rebuild the temporal points and sideburns/tendrils to complete the female hairline.

Basics of Hair Transplantation

The old "hair plugs" that once were used in hair transplantation are no longer. Plugs were grafts of hair, about the size of a pencil eraser, that were taken from the back of the head and transplanted on top of the head. In fact, they are as far from state-of-the-art medicine as the horse and buggy is from a Tesla Roadster. Modern transplanted hair is natural, refined, and matched to the direction, angle, and caliber of the hair it replaces or mimics. In modern hair transplantation, only single follicular units are used (as opposed to the "plug" grafts which contained multiple follicular units).

Follicular Unit

A *follicular unit,* known as an *FU,* is the anatomical unit of hair. It typically contains one to three hairs, as well as *sebaceous glands,* nerves, and a small muscle. The follicular unit grows as a tiny clump that can only be identified with a microscope. Hairs at the hairline contain only single-hair follicular units, resulting in a shadowing effect and a natural beginning to the hairline.

Harvesting these follicular units is particularly desirable for women's faces, where a soft frame is essential. The two- and three-haired follicular units are equally necessary, however, because they add to the hair's overall density and fullness. These characteristics are what make a woman's hair lushly amenable to styling.

During a modern hair transplant, follicular unit grafts are obtained in two ways. The first method, sometimes called *follicular unit transplant (FUT)* or "strip," involves taking a small linear strip of hair from the back of the head. Hair in this area is known as the *donor area,* and it is genetically immune to the hormones that cause pattern hair loss.

Follicular Unit Excision

The second method is to obtain grafts by shaving this donor area and taking the grafts out one at a time with a tiny circular "punch" that measures 1.2 mm. This is called *follicular unit excision (FUE),* and grafts obtained this way are

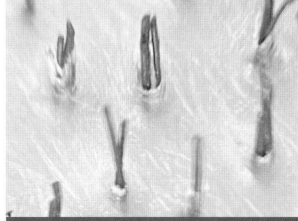

Naturally occurring units of hair—follicular units. Note that each graft is commonly comprised of either a single hair, two hairs, or three hairs.

more delicate and may grow poorly; some grafts may not survive.

The main advantage of the FUE approach is that it leaves only a pencil-thin scar, typically an advantage in those who prefer to wear their hair buzzed short. But for any patient who is planning to wear their hair longer than 1 cm, the linear method is preferred because it obtains more grafts that have a good chance for survival.

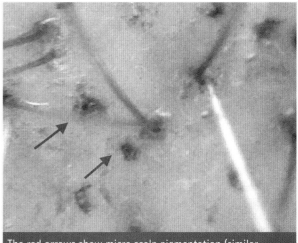

The red arrows show micro scalp pigmentation (similar to tattoos) as a camouflage technique that creates the appearance of hair shafts.

Hair Transplants after FFS

As mentioned earlier, much of what makes a woman's face instantly recognizable as female is the way in which her hair frames her face. So, in many cases, hair transplantation can improve facial feminization. However, it is wise to plan for hair transplantation after FFS. Wait for at least six months, or often nine to twelve months, after FFS before having hair transplants. Any scars from FFS should be healed. This healed tissue helps a hair transplant surgeon to get the best overall result in both hair density and the direction of hair growth.

With proper medication management (including finasteride, dutasteride, and minoxidil) and low-level light therapy, the time for new hair growth can be significantly improved. Also, if needed, follow-up grafting can be performed to create greater density and volume after the majority of the initial hair grafting shows growth —typically at about nine to twelve months later.

Hairline Feminization

Because female hairlines are so much lower than male hairlines, one of the first parts of fully feminizing the "frame" of the face is to perform a hairline-lowering procedure. Other than the obvious advantage of a lower hairline, this procedure simultaneously accomplishes several goals when done correctly.

First, it can remove tiny hairs that grow naturally at the edge of a hairline—leaving thicker and denser hair to frame of the face. Second, the incision reshapes the hairline. Third, the scarring is minimal, and can be nearly imperceptible. Thus, most well-done hairline-lowering procedures

Camouflage and Nonsurgical Options

Hair transplant surgery can sometimes be limited in what it can accomplish. If a patient does not have enough adequate grafts to achieve the patient's goals, nonsurgical options for camouflage are available.

HAIR FIBERS. Made of tiny bits of cotton or wool, hair fibers adhere to your natural hair. They can be sprinkled onto the hair and scalp, camouflaging thin or bald spots. They make fine hair appear thicker, and they stay in place regardless of a stiff breeze or a hand through the hair.

SCALP MICROPIGMENTATION (SMP). This camouflage technique is like a tattoo that creates tiny little dots of pigment just under the surface of the skin. These dots have the appearance of hairs and help cover bald spots. Made with a tiny needle, these pigments are subtle and layered to create a three-dimensional effect. Fading of the tiny dots does occur over time depending on one's exposure to UV light.

WIGS AND HAIRPIECES. For some patients with significant hair loss, hair transplants are not a solution. For these patients, a partial or full hairpiece can provide a seamless and fully functioning alternative. Often, a hairline can be transplanted to provide naturalness for a hairpiece behind it. Or the grafting and surgery are used to concentrate on adding as much density as possible to the frontal area, while a hairpiece is used to cover the vertex/crown. Full wigs can work well if hair is limited on the sides and at the back of the head.

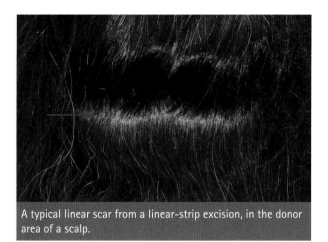

A typical linear scar from a linear-strip excision, in the donor area of a scalp.

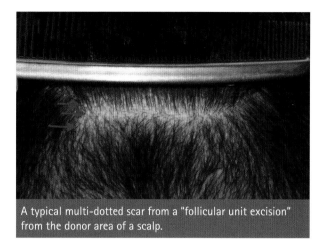

A typical multi-dotted scar from a "follicular unit excision" from the donor area of a scalp.

result in a dense hairline with thick hair and a negligible scar.

Unfortunately, not all hairline goals can be met with a hairline-lowering procedure alone. The extent of shaping is limited, usually to a curve shape. Because normal female hairlines have a high degree of curves and variation, a hairline shape that is achievable with incision alon, does not always mimic this natural irregularity.

In these cases, grafting with individual follicles is most useful. Like using a fine brush to add detail on a landscape canvas, single grafts are used to create a more feminine hairline.

Techniques for Feminizing the Hairline

In contrast to older techniques, modern hair transplantation with individual hair follicles almost always results in a very natural and dense appearance. Interestingly, hair loss only becomes noticeable when over 70 percent of the hair mass is gone. Nevertheless, women do have a higher standard for density in their hair than men, because more hair is needed to support various styling options. For this reason, many female patients will opt for additional hair transplantation to increase overall density.

There are several techniques for doing this:

- *Grafts can be added to feminize a hairline all on their own without any other cosmetic surgeries.*

- *Grafts can be added after a hairline-lowering procedure or facial feminization surgery.*

- *Grafts can be added during a hairline-lowering procedure or facial feminization surgery.*

Long-Term Planning for Hairline Maintenance

Hair that grows naturally on a trans woman's head will have a set of genes that express male pattern hair loss throughout the lifetime of the hair. Of course, not all of them experience hair loss. For those with a genetic makeup that favors hair loss, hormonal therapy alone during a transition may not stop the process entirely.

Use of Medications and Light Therapy

To that end, ongoing medical treatments for hair growth such as minoxidil (Rogaine), DHT blockers (finasteride or dutasteride), and low-level light therapy may be a good idea. Estrogen therapy and testosterone inhibition (whether surgical or hormonal) are also effective at slowing the progression.

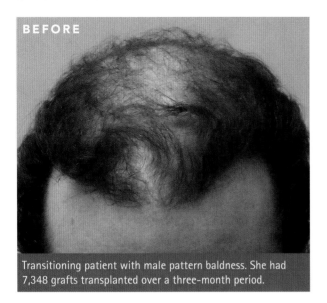

BEFORE

Transitioning patient with male pattern baldness. She had 7,348 grafts transplanted over a three-month period.

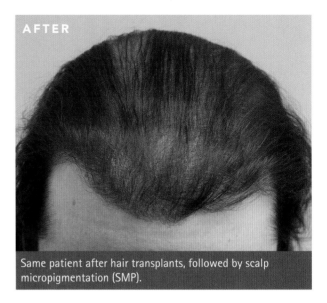

AFTER

Same patient after hair transplants, followed by scalp micropigmentation (SMP).

Plasma Injections

One of the newest treatments for hair loss is *platelet-rich plasma (PRP) therapy*. PRP uses the patient's blood to formulate a concentration of *platelets* (a type of blood cell) that are injected into the areas of hair loss. This therapy is still being studied, but it may reduce hair loss, thicken hair, and possibly lead to regrowth. Medicated shampoos (such as those made with ketoconazole, zinc, selenium, and coal tar) may also help.

Follow-Up Hair Transplants

If additional hair loss occurs, more hair replacement surgery may be needed. Because hair loss is by its very nature relentlessly progressive, hair restoration should be regarded as an ongoing process. It's a process that requires continued and long-term commitment to therapies that help with hair restoration. Luckily, many of the treatments we have, minimize the progression of hair loss.

Preparing for Your Hair Transplant Procedure

Patients are typically asked to abstain from alcohol or blood-thinning medications (such as ibuprofen and aspirin) for one to two weeks beforehand. Also, caffeine should be avoided on the day of surgery. For major surgeries, patients are asked to start fasting the night before; however, for hair transplants surgeries, patients are encouraged to eat a good breakfast. Then, patients are typically served lunch on the day of the hair transplant procedure. Note: If you're having other procedures, discuss fasting needs with your surgeon.

Undergoing Hair Transplant Surgery

For an uncomplicated hair transplant surgery, patients should expect to spend a full day in an outpatient surgery center or office-based operating room. Depending on the type of surgery (FUE or linear/FUT) being performed, certain areas of the head may be shaved.

Local Anesthesia

Full sedation in a hospital operating room with a hospital stay to recover is rarely necessary. Local anesthesia injections are given in the forehead and back of the head in what is known as a *ring block*, which lasts for the whole procedure.

Patients Encouraged to Relax During Procedure

Very few patients report discomfort during a hair transplant procedures. In fact, patients are made comfortable throughout the procedure. Typically, patients spend the day watching movies or listening to music while relaxing in the surgical chair. Patients are allowed to get up and move about for bathroom breaks.

Harvesting Hair Grafts

The *follicular unit excision (FUE)* technique, which takes hair grafts from the donor area at the back of the head, tends to produce fewer grafts than the linear method and is most commonly performed with a head that is shaved on the sides and back (but not necessarily on the top). Non-shaven FUE can be performed, but it may further limit the number of grafts because it takes longer to obtain high numbers. Grafts can live only six to eight hours outside the body before their survival starts to be compromised.

Scarring with either shaven or non-shaven FUE is diffuse and easy to camouflage with thousands of tiny scars that are roughly 1 mm in diameter. The linear technique tends to produce about 15–20 percent more grafts (2,500–3,500 grafts), and less overall scarring in terms of area (as measured in square centimeters). The shaved area is limited to the tissue being removed and can also simply be trimmed short instead of shaved. Thus, there is no delay while waiting for postoperative regrowth of hair in the donor area. Both surgeries produce scars that are well hidden within the hair and are even invisible with a formal "updo" hairstyle or short hairstyles. Either way, well-done hair transplants are nearly indistinguishable from natural native hair.

Recovery after Hair Transplant Procedure

After surgery, patients typically return to their home or hotel with a light headband-type bandage that absorbs any blood spotting in the donor area (a normal occurrence). There is usually no bandage on the grafted areas. Eating is not restricted, and medications are limited to pain control (either acetaminophen or narcotic as needed) and an antibiotic (usually three doses over twenty-four hours is sufficient).

Washing Hair the Next Morning

The morning after the surgery, the hair grafted area should be washed gently by first rinsing with water poured from a cup (to avoid the pressure of showerhead sprayers that may potentially dislodge the newly planted grafts). Then, any shampoo can be used to create a lather on the hands (baby shampoo or *zinc pyrithione* shampoo are suggested). The shampoo is then applied to the scalp with a gentle up-and-down patting motion. The grafts can be touched, just not rubbed sideways for the first three days after the surgery.

The reason for this caution is that any sideways motion can dislodge the grafts. A single dislodged graft is not a complete disaster because hundreds and even thousands are transplanted during a procedure. Yet, a dislodged graft can bleed profusely, which is frightening for the patient. If the graft is recovered and reinserted within a few hours, it has a 30 to 60 percent chance of regrowth, provided it is kept cold and wet until replacement. Complete rooting of the graft occurs at nine days post-surgery.

Washing the Donor Area

The donor area can be washed gently in the same manner as the graft area, but is much less susceptible to injury. Hair should be washed

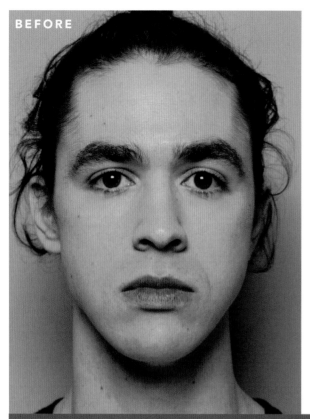
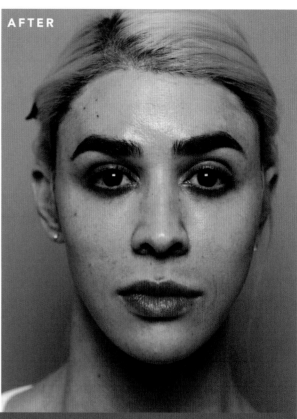

Before and after facial feminization surgery and hair transplants. FFS procedures included: Forehead Type III contouring, scalp advancement, brow lift, rhinoplasty, pan facial fat grafting, chin and jaw contouring, and thyroid cartilage reduction.

frequently—at least two to three times per day—for the first three days because moist wounds heal best. If hair is washed very frequently, the small crusts that commonly develop after transplantation are minimized and the transplanted areas return to normal much faster. Even if some crusts do form, they can be rubbed off starting on day four postoperatively. It is a good idea to rub them away because they are unsightly, a possible site of infection, and unnecessary for healing and growth. They also interfere with the application of minoxidil. So, if you are using minoxidil, wait about a week before applying it. Also, wait a week before using hairstyling products and camouflage products such as hair fibers.

How Transplanted Hair Grows

The short hairs that accompany the grafts during transplantation almost all fall out two to six weeks after surgery. This may seem disappointing, but it is a good sign. It means the hair follicle has taken root and the hair is going through its normal cycle of shedding, resting, and finally regrowth. Non-transplanted hair may shed temporarily as well, and this is termed *shock loss*. This incidence of shock loss is difficult to predict, and most cases are mild. Yet, there are some cases in which the loss is significant enough to cause a patient to think that "all their hair is falling out." This is not the case, and despite fears of complete baldness, the hair grows back.

New Hair Growth

New graft growth will appear at about six months and hairs will be short with a tapered end. The hair may initially be slightly curly or kinky, but this is temporary and usually gone after the first few haircuts. Full growth takes a year, and it is worth waiting for!

Wigs and hair extensions should be avoided almost completely after a transplant, because they are known to retard hair growth. If necessary, they can be worn for camouflage for no longer than a few (one to three) hours at a time starting about ten days after surgery.

Side Effects and Potential Complications

The incidence of infection is low and is usually limited to an occasional "ingrown hair" (technically an "inclusion cyst") in the donor area or the recipient zone. These usually happen within one to three months after surgery. Ingrown hairs occur in batches and can be easily treated with hot compresses, topical steroids, short courses of antibiotics, and simply "popping" any of the little pimple-like eruptions. Temporary numbness of the scalp can also be a complication but resolves in almost every case within a few months.

Commonly Asked Questions

How are grafts obtained in a modern hair transplant? In the *follicular unit transplant (FUT)*, a small linear strip of hair is taken from the back of the head, called the donor area. Grafts can also be obtained by shaving the donor area and taking the grafts out one at a time with a small circular punch, a method called *follicular unit excision (FUE)*. Both techniques can produce excellent results.

What can a surgical hairline lowering procedure accomplish? Besides lowering the hairline to appear more like a female, this surgery also can remove miniaturized hair at the end of a hairline. As a result, thicker and denser hair will frame the face. The scarring after recovery is typically a fine line along the edge of the hair.

Yet, not all hairline goals can be accomplished through this surgery. The shaping during this procedure does not have the high degree of curves and variation found in the typical female hairline. So, grafting with individual hair follicles during surgery can help achieve a natural feminine hairline shape. Still, many patients undergoing facial feminization will opt for additional hair transplantation to achieve the density needed for feminine hairstyles.

Why is a long-term plan needed to create and maintain feminine hair? Hormonal therapy during a transition can reduce hair loss, but it doesn't always stop it entirely. Thus, treatments such as medications like minoxidil (Rogaine), finasteride (Propecia), and low-level light therapy may be needed to maintain female hair growth and reduce hair loss over time. If you are genetically prone to baldness, more hair replacement surgery may also be needed after your initial procedure to reduce hair loss. After all, hair loss is often progressive as we age. Luckily, today's treatments are quite effective for minimizing such hair loss.

A Final Note

A female hairline is crucial to feminizing the face. During your transition, you can feminize the hairline through both surgical and nonsurgical approaches. However, you also need a long-term plan for maintaining the feminine characteristics of your hair and hairline, because hair changes over time.

Modern hair transplantation is one way to feminize the face and reduce male pattern hair loss.

Another approach is to lower the hairline with a facial feminization procedure and add additional hair grafts during or after the procedure.

If these options don't achieve your goals, products made of tiny hair fibers or hair-like fibers can be used to camouflage thin areas or bald spots. Wigs and partial wigs can also be used for the same purpose, especially if you have large areas of hair loss. Scalp pigmentation is also a good camouflage technique that creates tiny dots of pigment just under the skin, mimicking the appearance of increased hair density at the microscopic level.

The trick to having any of these techniques be effective is to find an experienced and artistic practitioner—one who can closely match your goals and work with you throughout the entire process.

Appendix A
Specialized Surgical Training and Board Certification

IN ORDER TO BE SAFE and competent performing the complicated facial feminization procedures described in this book, your surgeon should have completed formal training in all of the following three areas of surgery:

- *plastic surgery*
- *formal jaw surgery training (maxillofacial or orthognathic surgery)*
- *a formal craniofacial fellowship at a major teaching hospital*

The purpose of this appendix is to provide expanded information on selecting the right experienced surgeon for your procedures. The information in this appendix may prevent you from ending up with a serious "bad outcome" from your surgery.

Before a surgeon undertakes to learn any of the three specialties identified above, that person must have surgical training.

That statement appears almost totally obvious. And it should be obvious. However, there are practitioners claiming on the internet and at transgender conferences to be "FFS surgeons" who were never formally or properly trained as surgeons.

Dr. Ousterhout initially followed a career path in dentistry. He followed up by extensive training in maxillofacial surgery. Maxillofacial surgery includes the field of "jaw surgery." But, it became apparent to him that even that level of training was inadequate for his goals. So, he acquired a medical degree and then further trained in general and plastic surgery. After that, he went to Paris to train in the then new field of craniofacial surgery.

Dr. Deschamps-Braly trained in surgery and plastic surgery. Then he was admitted to one of the rare craniofacial surgery fellowship programs in the United States. Afterward, he traveled to Paris and Zurich where he pursued still more advanced training in craniofacial surgery, aesthetic surgery of the face, and *orthognathic (jaw)* surgery.

According to Dr. Deschamps-Braly, although we followed different paths in our surgical training, we both ultimately ended up at the same place: fully trained in all three of the essential surgical specialties required to perform FFS properly.

A growing number of patients now seek us out for "redos" of their previous facial surgeries originally performed by other surgeons. It has not escaped our notice that almost all of the "redo" requests come from patients whose original procedures were performed by surgeons who were not formally trained in craniofacial surgery.

Plastic Surgery

Short History of Plastic Surgery

Most people think of plastic surgery from the perspective of TV reality shows, facelifts, or breast implants. However plastic surgery was first described in writing around 600 BCE. As a diverse surgical specialty, plastic surgery not only overlaps with other disciplines of medicine, but also merges medical science with the art of physical and aesthetic restoration.

During and immediately after World War I, the field of facial plastic surgery rapidly evolved to address the large number of facial disfigurements that resulted from that terrible conflict. Likewise, many hundreds of thousands of children with cleft lips and cleft palates have now had their lives restored by skilled plastic surgeons.

Why Is Plastic Surgery Important to You?

The surgical skill sets required to properly perform facial feminization surgery start with formal plastic surgery training. That is the foundation. To that foundation, a surgeon who

aspires to perform consistently safe and successful FFS must then take the time and have the devotion required to acquire two additional surgical skill sets: jaw (orthognathic/maxillofacial) surgery and craniofacial surgery.

Orthognathic Surgery

Short History of Orthognathic Surgery

Orthognathic surgery is a technical name for a group of surgical procedures that can change the shape and location of the upper (maxilla) and lower (mandible) jaws. It is easier to just call it "jaw surgery." In its modern form, jaw surgery consists of a relatively recent set of surgical procedures that were largely developed in Switzerland by Dr. Obwegeser around the same time that Dr. Paul Tessier developed craniofacial surgery.

The figure right (A1-1) is a digital planning model created by Dr. Deschamps-Braly for one of his patients that illustrates the dramatic changes possible in a patient's maxilla (upper jaw) in the hands of a skilled jaw surgeon.

Over the years, some dentists have also trained in what is termed *maxillofacial surgery*. Normally, maxillofacial surgery training includes all of the procedures involved in the description of "orthognathic" surgery. But maxillofacial training does not include the broader set of surgical training and skills involved in either plastic surgery or craniofacial surgery.

This distinction is important to keep in mind as you evaluate the qualifications of your prospective FFS surgeon. Dentists trained in maxillofacial surgery are not qualified as either plastic surgeons or as craniofacial surgeons. Unfortunately, there are some dental practitioners with maxillofacial training who inappropriately market themselves to prospective FFS patients.

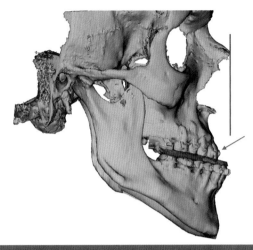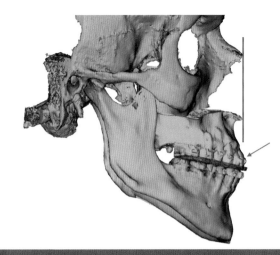

Figure A1-1 Digital virtual surgical planning in orthognathic (jaw) surgery.

Every plastic surgeon gets some passing exposure to "jaw surgery" during their surgical residency training. But that limited exposure during their formal surgical residency is not sufficient for those surgeons to be competent in performing the complex jaw surgeries involved in FFS.

Why Is Jaw Surgery Important to You?

A surgeon's formal specialized jaw surgery training is important to you if you are undergoing FFS. Without that training, your surgeon will not be capable of properly evaluating what can be done for your facial architecture. Nor can the surgeon safely and consistently alter the contour and shape of your jaw and chin in FFS surgery.

Surgeons without adequate jaw surgery training may advise patients that they "really do not need" significant jaw contouring or surgery for facial feminization. As an alternative, the surgeon may recommend implants when jaw surgery would be safer and most appropriate. Even more of a problem is the surgeon who is not properly trained to do jaw surgeries but does them anyway.

Craniofacial Surgery

Short History of Craniofacial Surgery

The field of craniofacial surgery was invented by Dr. Paul Tessier in Paris, during the 1960s and early 1970s. During the 1950s, Dr. Tessier first located and then studied numerous skulls from children who had died due to congenital facial deformities. He sometimes conducted postmortem practice surgery on some of those skulls and learned to reassemble the pieces to correct the problems that had caused the early deaths. Dr. Tessier then developed surgical techniques that allowed him to reshape the bony pieces of a child's skull and reassemble them to transform the head and face of a child. In this way, he corrected their deformities.

For those children it was a miracle, as they could thereafter live a relatively normal life. In other cases, the craniofacial surgeon will completely remodel the skull of an infant or small child afflicted with *craniosynostosis*. In children with this condition, the bony growth plates in their heads are prematurely fused and fail to grow to accommodate their rapidly growing brains. Without lifesaving craniofacial surgery, the child will not survive. In the surgery, large portions of the bone structure of the forehead and cranial vault are removed in the operating room and reshaped and reconfigured. The new bone structure is then reimplanted in the child to enlarge the cranial volume of the head so that the brain has room to grow normally.

Why is that skill set important to you? Only a surgeon with expert training and experience in craniofacial surgery can safely and comfortably perform the demanding surgery required to transform the face of a transgender patient. Dr. Deschamps-Braly is presently the last American surgeon to have traveled to Paris in order to complete a fellowship in craniofacial surgery with one of the early pioneers in that field: Dr. Daniel Marchac. Unfortunately, Dr. Marchac has passed away. Only with the knowledge, experience, and skills developed from years of performing intricate and complex craniofacial surgeries was Dr. Ousterhout able to develop the specific procedures required for FFS surgeries.

Dr. Deschamps-Braly has very recently pioneered and performed what is believed to be the first pediatric craniofacial surgeries using modern techniques for digital "virtual" surgeries and 3-D custom-printed surgical templates. The results have been outstanding.

Because the number of trained craniofacial surgeons is so small, at present there is no board certification in this very specialized field. So be wary of surgeons who claim to have been trained in this specialty when they have not.

Why Is Craniofacial Surgery Important to You?

Every patient is different, and every patient's individual soft tissue and bone structure has the potential to surprise the surgeon during surgery.

There are many unusual conditions that can arise during feminization surgery of the face and particularly the forehead. Only a surgeon trained in craniofacial surgery will be able to address and correct those issues as they occasionally arise, almost always unexpectedly.

Rigorous, formal academic training in craniofacial surgery and then subsequent extensive hands-on operating room training in all aspects of FFS surgery are essential for your surgeon. This training is crucial for consistently, safely, and successfully feminizing the forehead.

The internet reveals a growing number of facial feminization surgeons who have dental surgery training backgrounds, and in some cases suggest they were trained in "craniofacial" surgery. This "confusion" is caused by the fact that sometimes "maxillofacial" surgery programs use the name "cranio-maxillofacial" in the name. If you see the use of that variation on the term "maxillofacial surgeon" you should understand that description does not include the much more extensive training of a craniofacial surgeon.

When I (Dr. Ousterhout) began to perform the first FFS cases, I followed Dr. Tessier's earlier example with children. In my case, I located a large collection of young and mature adult male and female skulls in a "skull collection" at an academic facility. Then, I studied those skulls in detail in order to understand precisely how to successfully alter the face of a man to that of a woman. After working as an assistant to Dr. Deschamps-Braly for over two years and after many surgeries, that knowledge gained from my earlier studies has now been secured for a new generation.

Surgeons Who Claim to Do "Everything"

Most surgeons focus their expertise on one or two specific areas of specialization involving limited portions of the human anatomy. Experience has established that this practice has great benefits for patients. However, some surgeons attempt to perform many completely different surgical procedures involving multiple different parts of the human anatomy.

Common sense suggests that having expertise in everything would be rare or, frankly, impossible.

Facial feminization is very different and much more complex than traditional soft tissue cosmetic surgery. Please do not accept that surgeons who advertise and perform a laundry list of virtually every plastic surgery procedure will also be skilled at remodeling your facial bone structure. There are surgeons who claim to do FFS surgeries, but when you look at the surgeon's advertised "practice profile," the surgeon claims to be competent in doing everything from tummy tucks to Brazilian butt-lifts to cosmetic vein stripping. Do you really want to rely on that surgeon to remodel the bony structure of your face?

Check Surgeon Credentials

So how do you decide whether your surgeon has the right training background to pick up a sharp knife and work on your face? For starters, you need to review the doctor's credentials to make sure the doctor has the training, experience, and ability to safely perform your surgery. Look for solid evidence in your surgeon's biography and credentials to confirm completion of all the essential education and training.

Finally, do not assume that every equally trained surgeon has the same ability to create a stellar result. They do not. Producing a feminine version of a masculine face takes years of specialized training, experience, patience, unusual skill, and, yes, artistry.

The next section about board certification will explain how you can check your prospective surgeon's credentials.

Board Certification

What is board certification? Board certification is a formal statement by a legitimate organization of specially trained medical professionals that a candidate doctor has successfully met a rigorous set of educational, training, and experience requirements. Legitimate "board certification" involves a rather lengthy process during which a highly trained and experienced candidate surgeon is required to pass a series of detailed written tests. Then later, after being in practice, a candidate surgeon must submit complete case files on a number of the candidate surgeon's patients for review. These case files are viewed by independent surgeons and the candidate surgeon must pass an oral exam and answer questions about the surgeries performed.

We place serious emphasis on the use of the word "legitimate" when we write about board certification. There are some "board certifications" that do not meet the rigorous requirements we have described. Many of them are simply "vanity" board certifications. With rare exceptions, a vanity board certification is one that is not sanctioned and recognized by the American Board of Medical Specialties, often referred to simply as the ABMS (www.abms.org). There is a similar organization in Europe—the Union Européenne des Médecins Spécialistes (UEMS; www.uems.eu). For many decades, the ABMS has approved and recognized "board certifications" in various specialty areas. At present, the ABMS sanctions and recognizes a total of twenty-four medical specialties. These twenty-four specialties cover the entire range of medical science.

Only one of those twenty-four medical specialties is relevant to the field of facial feminization surgery. If your physician is not board certified by the American Board of Plastic Surgery (ABPS: www.abplasticsurgery.org), we would strongly suggest that you reconsider your choice. The American Board of Plastic Surgery (ABPS) is an ABMS-sanctioned board. This certification is what your U.S. or Canadian surgeon should have. For example, the American Board of Cosmetic Surgery (ABCS) is not an ABMS-sanctioned board. You should not accept this certification in your surgeon. The American Board of Facial Plastic Surgery (ABFPS) is also not an ABMS-sanctioned board.

The above examples are just two of the many "boards" that are not recognized and sanctioned by the ABMS. The standards for admission to many of the "vanity" boards are seldom anywhere near as stringent as those for an ABMS-sanctioned board. Physicians who advertise affiliation with some "cosmetic surgery boards" may have only completed one or two years of training after medical school.

By contrast, a typical plastic surgeon who is board certified by the American Board of Plastic Surgery, will have completed a minimum of five years of intense and focused training after medical school. Often, they will have also completed still further specialized training.

The more any doctor or friend tries to convince you that any one of the vanity board certifications is "equal to" or the same as a board certification sanctioned by the ABMS—the more strongly you should reconsider any decision you may have made to select that surgeon for your needs.

Again, in the United States and Canada, the relevant board certification is the American Board of Plastic Surgery (ABPS) at www.abplasticsurgery.org. The sponsoring organization is the American Board of Medical Specialties (www.abms.org).

How do you verify which board certification is genuine and not a "vanity" board certification? Fortunately, in North America, that is easy. Simply go to www.certificationmatters.org and fill in the name of any surgeon you are considering. If the surgeon is not board certified by the American Board of Plastic Surgery (ABPS) then you should reevaluate your search for a suitable surgeon.

In Europe, the legitimate board certifications are sponsored by the European Union of Medical Specialties (UEMS, Union Européenne des Médecins Spécialistes; www.uems.eu). For facial feminization surgery, the relevant board certification is the European Board of Plastic Reconstructive and Aesthetic Surgery (EBOPRAS; www.ebopras.eu).

The search function at EBOPRAS allows you to check and see if your surgeon is a member of EBOPRAS. Your European surgeon's website should also clearly identify your surgeon as being certified by the EBOPRAS.

At present, within Europe, we are aware of only one surgeon who specializes in facial feminization and appears on the membership list of EBOPRAS. However, that can always change—so you should check the website and see if your surgeon is in fact, board certified.

Unfortunately, the situation in the rest of the world (outside of the United States, Canada, Europe, and the former commonwealth countries) is more difficult. There are no organizations in Asia, Latin or South America, Korea, or other places that have the authority of the long-standing medical specialty organizations in the United States and Europe.

Board Certification Is a Necessary Part of the Qualification Process, But It Is Not the Whole Picture

While obtaining the necessary training and experience to successfully pass certification board exams, a surgeon will likely have also pursued other specialized training. For example, because the specialty is so small, there are no "board certifications" for craniofacial surgeons. A surgeon interested in the field can apply for a fellowship in one of the limited number of teaching hospital–based craniofacial programs. If accepted, the surgeon will spend a full year doing craniofacial surgery under the supervision of a highly experienced craniofacial surgeon.

A surgeon not already fully trained in jaw surgery can, likewise, pursue a fellowship in jaw surgery. There should be formal certificates or other documentation that establish that a surgeon has successfully accomplished their fellowship training in the additional specialty fields. Normally, those certificates, if they exist, will in this internet age be visible somewhere on the surgeon's website. If you do not find them there, then that is a reason to make further inquiries.

Admitting Privileges: Office-Based and Freestanding Surgery Facilities

Sometimes a surgeon may propose to reduce the cost of your surgery by using an office-based or ambulatory surgery center. Under the

right circumstances, those facilities may offer an appropriate level of care and also an attractive price.

Both types of facilities have advantages and disadvantages. Which type of facility is your surgeon performing your surgery at, should be a question you should ask.

Hospitals offer the safety of a highly regulated environment with lots of resources should something not go well. However, hospitals significantly increase the cost of care.

Surgery centers on the other hand, may offer cost advantages in many cases so long as you can ensure that the surgery center your surgeon is operating in, is accredited by one of the governing bodies that regulates ambulatory surgical centers (ASCs).

In addition, for facial feminization surgery, it is often necessary to keep patients one night in the facility. You need to make sure that the facility that your surgeon uses allows for overnight stays with adequate nursing care.

Your surgeon, regardless of where he/she performs your surgery, should maintain hospital privileges in case your care needs to be transferred to a hospital at some point during your medical care. It is imperative that your surgeon should have admitting privileges to a "local" hospital and not just any hospital. The hospital should be relatively close to the ambulatory surgery center if that is where your surgery is scheduled to occur. The last thing you want, is for your surgeon to send you to the hospital under the care of someone else because he/she doesn't have hospital privileges.

Appendix B
Commonly Asked Questions

My surgeon trained on the continent in maxillofacial surgery, and says he also trained in craniofacial surgery. Isn't that good enough?

Based on your description, your surgeon should be board certified by the European Board of Oro-Maxillo-Facial Surgery (www.ebomfs.eu). As this book goes to print, that board's website does not have a useful search function for non-members to see if a surgeon really is truly board certified. If you go to the surgeon's web pages, then the surgeon should clearly state that the surgeon is board certified by the EBOMFS and provide the details.

Keep in mind, every surgeon who is, in fact, certified by one of the recognized board certification organizations, will display that fact on their website.

After you establish that your European surgeon is actually board certified by the EBOMFS, then determine if your surgeon really was further trained in both plastic and craniofacial surgery. A statement on a surgeon's website that your surgeon is a "cranio-maxillofacial" surgeon does

not mean he or she was trained in craniofacial surgery.

My surgeon says he is "triple" board certified. Isn't that sufficient?

No. In fact, that sort of claim is a virtual "red flag" that the surgeon is relying upon membership in one or more of the "vanity" boards to embellish their presentation on the internet. If your surgeon is in the United States or Canada, go to www.certificationmatters.org and find out if the surgeon is a member of the American Board of Plastic Surgery (ABPS) at www.abplasticsurgery.org.

If not, you should probably continue your search for another surgeon to transform your face. If your surgeon is board certified by the ABPS, then do further research to establish that they are also trained in jaw surgery and craniofacial surgery.

My surgeon says he is board certified by one of the boards in a country in Latin America. I cannot afford surgery with one of the surgeons in the United States. What is the risk?

You are in a very unfortunate situation. It is extremely difficult to evaluate the legitimate qualifications of a surgeon who is trained outside the North American/Western European/English commonwealth environment. If you cannot raise the money for your surgery from savings, family, or loans, then you might consider delaying your surgery until you can afford to get it done properly.

We realize that is not an answer you may want to hear. However, the reality is that we see far too many patients in our office seeking "redo" surgeries because the original surgeon was not properly trained, certified, and qualified.

As a result, the final total cost to "get it right," is always substantially more than it would have been by selecting an appropriate initial surgeon.

My surgeon lists his membership in several different medical groups with a lot of impressive titles and websites. Is that the same as being "board" certified?

Good question. The answer is "no." It is often relatively easy to "sign up" and pay your annual dues and be a member of any number of medical societies.

Do not be overly impressed by a long list of mere "memberships."

Bibliography

Books and Selected Applicable Publications by Douglas Ousterhout M.D., D.D.S.

Books

Aesthetic Contouring of the Craniofacial Skeleton, Ousterhout DK., ed. Boston MA: Little, Brown and Company; 1991.

Facial Feminization Surgery: A Guide for the Trangendered Woman, Ousterhout DK., Omaha, NE: Addicus Books Inc; 2009.

Selected Articles and Publications

Ousterhout DK, Baker S, Zlotolow I. Methylmethacrylate onlay implants in the treatment of forehead deformities secondary to craniosynostosis. *J Maxillofac Surg.* 1980; 8:228-33.

Ousterhout DK, Penoff, J. Surgical treatment of facial deformity secondary to acromegaly. *Ann Plast Surg.* 1981; 7 (1): 69-74.

Ousterhout DK, Weill R. The role of the lateral canthal tendon in lower eyelid laxity. *Plast Reconstr Surg.* 1982; 69: 620-22.

Ousterhout DK, Vargervik K, Miller A. Nasal airway as it relates to the timing of the mid and lower facial osteotomies. *Annals of Plastic Surgery.* 1983: 11 (3): 175-82.

Ousterhout DK. Clinical experience in cranial and facial reconstruction with demineralized bone: A preliminary report. *Plastic Surgery Forum VI.* 1983: 50-52.

Ousterhout DK. Clinical experience in cranial and facial reconstruction with demineralized bone. *Ann Plast Surg.* 1985; 15: 367-73.

Ousterhout DK. Facial disfigurement: Physical and psychological aspects from a surgeon's perspective. *Body and Mind: Emotional Problems in Physical Disabilities.* The Mind and Medicine Symposia Series. University of California, San Francisco; 1985: 31-34.

Edwards MS, Ousterhout DK. The use of autogenous skull bone grafts to reconstruct large and/or complex skull defects in children and adolescents. *J Neurosurg.* 1987; 20: 273-280.

Melsen B, Ousterhout DK. Anatomy and development of the pterygopalatomaxillary region, studied in relation to LeFort osteotomies. *Ann. Plast. Surg.* 1987; 19: 16-28.

Ousterhout DK. Feminization of the forehead, contour changing to improve female aesthetics. *Plast Reconstr Surg.* 1987; 79: 701-711.

Ousterhout DK, Vargervik K. Surgical treatment of the jaw deformities in hemi facial microsomia. *Aust NZ J Surg.* 1987; 57: 77-87.

Ousterhout DK, Vargervik, K. Aesthetic improvement resulting from craniofacial surgery in craniosynostosis syndromes. *J Craniomaxillofac. Surg.* 1987; 15: 171-232.

Vargervick K, Farias M, Ousterhout DK. Changing in zygomatic arch position following experimental lateral displacement. *J Craniomaxillofac Surg.* 1987; 15: 208-212.

Ousterhout DK, Melsen B. Timing and placement of the posterior maxillary osteotomy in LeFort procedures on the basis of anatomy and development. In: Marchac D, ed. *Craniofacial Surgery.* Springer-Verlag GmbH; 1987: 170-179.

Zlotolow IM, Ousterhout DK, Methylmethacrylate forehead onlay implants in the treatment of upper facial deformities. *Maxillofac Prosthet.* 1987; 10: 18-24.

Ousterhout DK, Vargervik K, Tomer B, et al. Post-traumatic condylar hyperplasia. *Ann Plast Surg.* 1989; 22: 163-172.

Ousterhout DK. Feminizing the skull. In: Marsh J, ed. *Current Therapy in Plastic and Reconstructive Surgery, Head and Neck.* Toronto, Canada: Decker; 1989: 483-491.

Ousterhout DK, Vargervick K. Orthognathic Surgery. In: Lehman J, ed. Retrognathism. *Clin Plast Surg.* 1989; 4: 687-693.

Ousterhout DK, Zlotolow IM. Aesthetic improvement of the forehead utilizing methylmethacrylate onlay implants. *Aesthetic Plast Surg.* 1990; 14: 281-286.

Ousterhout DK. Combined suction-assisted lipectomy, surgical lipectomy, and surgical abdominoplasty. *Ann Plast Surg.* 1990; 24: 126.

Ousterhout DK. Mandibular angle augmentation and reduction. In: Whitaker, LA, ed. *Clinics in Plastic Surgery: Aesthetic Surgery of the Facial Skeleton,* Philadelphia, PA: WB Saunders Co.; 1991: 153-162.

Ousterhout DK. The forehead: Its relationship to nasal aesthetics, indications for and methods of Contour Changing. In: Gruber RP, Peck GC, eds. *Rhinoplasty: State of the Art.* St. Louis, MO: CV Mosby Co.; 1991.

Ritter EF, Moelleken BRK, Mathes SJ, Ousterhout, DK. The course of the inferior alveolar neurovascular canal in relation to sliding genioplasty. *J Craniofac Surg.* 1992; 3 (1): 20-24.

Ousterhout DK. Supraorbital Rim and Forehead Implant. In: Hinderer UT, ed. *Plastic Surgery.* Volume 1. Lectures and Panels. International Congress Series 935. 1992: 441-444.

Ousterhout DK. Aesthetic contouring of the upper face. In: McNamara JA, ed. *Aesthetics and the Treatment of Facial Form.* Volume 28, Craniofacial Growth Series. Center for Human Growth and Development. The University of Michigan, Ann Arbor, Michigan. 1993: 147-167.

Lykins, CL, Friedman CD, Ousterhout DK. Polymeric implants in craniomaxillofacial reconstruction. In: Friedman CD, Constantino PD, guest eds. Craniofacial Skeletal Augmentation and Replacement. *The Otolaryngologic Clinics of North America.* 1994: 1015.

Ousterhout DK. Sliding genioplasty, avoiding mental nerve injuries. In: Marchac D, ed. *Craniofacial Surgery #6.* Bologna, Italy: Monduzzi Editore; 1995: 315-316.

Ousterhout DK, Stelnicki E. Prevention of thermal tissue injury induced by the application of polymethylmethacrylate to the calvarium. *J Craniofac Surg.* 1996: 7 (3): 192-195.

Ousterhout DK, Stelnicki E. Plastic surgery's plastic. *Clin Plast Surg.* 1996; 23: 183-190.

Ousterhout DK. Sliding genioplasty, avoiding mental nerve injuries. *J Craniofac Surg.* 1996; 7: 298.

Ousterhout DK. Reconstruction of cranial vault defects with methylmethacrylate. *J Craniofac Surg.* 1996; 7: 483.

Ousterhout DK. Prevention of mental nerve injuries and masculinization of the chin by osteotomies. In: Chen Yu-Ray, ed. *Craniofacial Surgery. #8.* Bologna, Italy: Monduzzi; 1999: 341-343.

Ousterhout DK. Aesthetic contouring of the bony forehead. In: Terino EO, Flowers RS. *The Art of Allplastic Facial Contouring.* St. Louis, MO: Mosby; 2000: 67-76.

Ousterhout DK. Forehead contouring with methylmethacrylate. Operative Techniques. *Plast Reconstr Surg.* 2003; 9: 53-58.

Ousterhout DK. Feminization of the chin: A review of 385 consecutive cases. In: Salyer K, ed. *Craniofacial Surgery.* Medimond International Proceeding (Bologna, Italy); 2003: 461-463.

Ousterhout DK. Feminization of the mandibular body: A review of 688 consecutive cases. In David DJ, ed. *Craniofacial Surgery*, #11. Medimond International Proceeding (Bologna, Italy); 2005: 135-137.

Ousterhout DK. Paul Tessier and facial skeletal masculinization. *Ann Plast Surg.* 2011; 67 (6): S10-S15.

Textbook and Selected Applicable Publications by Jordan Deschamps-Braly, MD:

Deschamps-Braly J, Black JS, Denny A. Advantages of calvarial vault distraction for the late treatment of cephalocranial disproportion. *J Craniofac Surg.* 2016; 27 (6): 1505. Presenting Author. International Society of Craniofacial Surgeons Biennial Congress, Japan (2015).

Deschamps-Braly J, Sun P, Ousterhout DK. Virtual planning of forehead surgery for craniosynostosis. Presented: Annual Meeting Pan American Craniofacial Society, Puerto Vallarta, Mexico. March, 2015.

Ousterhout DK, Deschamps-Braly J. Facial feminization surgery. Presentation. Visiting Professors—Yale University.

Deschamps-Braly J. Facial feminization surgery. Orthognathic surgery. Visiting Professor—University of Oklahoma Grand Rounds.

Deschamps-Braly J. Facial feminization surgery for the young transsexual. UCSF Benioff Children's Hospital Oakland Pediatric Grand Rounds.

Deschamps-Braly J. Neonatal distraction of craniofacial skeleton for airway restriction. UCSF Benioff Children's Hospital Oakland. Pediatric Grand Rounds.

Deschamps-Braly J. Craniofacial surgery and application to common neonatal conditions, Part I & Part II. California Pacific Medical Center Pediatric Grand Rounds.

Hettinger P, Deschamps-Braly J, Denny A. Volumetric analysis of airway and mandible after neonatal distraction. Presented: International Society of Craniofacial Surgery: Jackson Hole Wyoming. Sept. 14, 2013.

Beidas OE, Deschamps-Braly J, Morgan AM, et al. Safety and efficacy of recombinant human bone morphogenetic protein 2 on cranial defect closure in the pediatric population. *J Craniofac Surg.* 2013; 24(3): 917–922. doi:10.1097/SCS.0b013e318256657c.

Deschamps-Braly J. Craniosynostosis and cranial volume: Indications and considerations. Visiting Guest Lecture: University Hospital Zurich.

Deschamps-Braly J. Use of vascularized bone graft with nitinol staples for treatment of non-union of the scaphoid. Presented: American Association for Hand Surgery: Las Vegas, NV. January 11, 2012.

Marchac D, Sati S, Renier D, Deschamps-Braly J, Marchac A. Hypertelorism correction: What happens with growth? Evaluation of a series of 95 surgical cases. *Plast Reconstr Surg.* 2012; 129(3): 713–727. doi:10.1097/PRS.0b013e3182402db1

Deschamps-Braly, J. Efficacy of rhBMP-2 on cranial defect closure in a pediatric population. Presented: International Society of Craniofacial Surgeons Biennial Meeting XIV Livingstone, Africa: Submitted to Journal of Craniofacial Surgery.

Deschamps-Braly, J. Volumetric analysis of cranial vault distraction for cephalocranial disproportion. Presented: International Society of Craniofacial Surgeons Biennial Meeting XIV Livingstone, Africa.

Deschamps-Braly J, Hettinger P, el Amm C, Denny AD. Volumetric analysis of cranial vault distraction for cephalocranial disproportion. *Pediatr Neurosurg.* 2011; 47(6): 396–405. doi:10.1159/000337873.

D'Andrea L A, Deschamps-Braly J, et al. Outcome of mandibular lengthening for infants with Pierre-Robin Sequence and upper airway obstruction. In: *SLEEP.* Vol. 34. Westchester, Il: Amer Acad Sleep Medicine.

Denny A. Deschamps-Braly J. Obstructive apnea in infants with Pierre Robin Sequence associated with impaired neurocognitive development. Poster Presentation 2011 Annual Sleep Association Meeting.

Deschamps-Braly J. Presented: NOE fractures and treatment. Wisconsin Foundations in

Craniomaxillofacial Surgery Course. Madison, Wisconsin.

El Amm CA, Deschamps-Braly JC, Workman MC, Knotts CC, Sawan KT. Midface buttress framework reconstruction after close-range high-energy injury. *Plast Reconstr Surg.* 2010; 126(6): 302e–304e. doi:10.1097/PRS.0b013e3181f63f7b.

Deschamps-Braly J. Sawan K, Manson, P. Decision making in isolated orbital roof fractures with case report of upper eyelid approach to treatment. *Plast Reconstr Surg.* 2010; 126(6): 308e–309e. doi:10.1097/PRS.0b013e3181f63f2a.

Deschamps-Braly J. Use of vascularized bone graft with nitinol staples for treatment of non-union of the scaphoid. Presented: American Association of Plastic Surgeons. 89th Annual Meeting. San Antonio, TX.

Deschamps-Braly J. Treatment of dynamic and static nasal tip deficiency. Presented: American Society of Plastic Surgeons Senior Residents.

Nusbaum B, Fuentefria S. Naturally Occurring Female Hairline Patterns, *Dermatol Surg.* 2009; 35: 907-913.

Unger WP, Shapiro RS, editors. *Hair Transplantation.* New York: Marcel Dekker, Inc.; 2004. P. 151-63.

Workman M, Deschamps-Braly J, Morgan A, Sawan K. Bidirectional barbed suture migration: A unique complication after intracuticular closure. *Aesthetic Plast Surg.* 2011; 35(4): 672–673. doi:10.1007/s00266-010-9644-1.

Hromadka M, Deschamps-Braly J, Sawan K, Amm el C. Delayed development of toxic shock syndrome following abdominal tissue expansion in a pediatric reconstruction patient. *Ann Plast Surg.* 2010; 64(2): 254–257. doi:10.1097/SAP.0b013e31819ff208.

Knotts CD, Morgan AL, Deschamps-Braly JC, Sawan KT, El Amm CA. "Mulching" integra for glans penis reconstruction. *Plast Reconstr Surg.* 2010; 126(3): 152e. doi:10.1097/PRS.0b013e3181e3b599.

Cranial bone graft to dorsum of nose 25 years later. Working Title—*In Preparation*, Dr. Mehdi Adham, Senior Author. Deschamps-Braly, J. Author.

Ahmad N, Lyles J, Panchal J, Deschamps-Braly J. Outcomes and complications based on experience with resorbable plates in pediatric craniosynostosis Patients. *J Craniofac Surg.* 2008; 19(3): 855–860. doi:10.1097/SCS.0b013e31816ae358.

Other References

Nusbaum B, Fuentefria S. Naturally occurring female hairline patterns, *Dermatol Surg* 2009; 35: 907-913.

Unger WP, Shapiro RS, editors *Hair Transplantation.* New York: Marcel Dekker, Inc.; 2004. P. 163.

Wang TT, Wessels L, Hussain G, et al. Discriminative thresholds in facial asymmetry: A review of the literature. *Aesthet Surg J.* 2017; 37 (4): 375-385.

Resources

Health

Trans Lifeline
translifeline.org
Crisis and suicide prevention hotline.

WPATH – World Professional Association of Transgender Health
wpath.org
Largest professional association focused on trans healthcare.

GLMA
glma.org
Organization committed to ensuring health equity for lesbian, gay, bisexual, transgender, queer (LGBTQ) and all sexual and gender minority (SGM) individuals, and equality for LGBTQ/SGM health professionals.

GATE
gate.ngo
Trans, gender diverse, and intersex advocacy in action.

Center of Excellence for Transgender Health
transhealth.ucsf.edu
San Francisco-based health resources.

FORGE
forge-forward.org
FORGE reduces the impact of trauma on trans/non-binary survivors and communities by empowering service providers, advocating for systems reform, and connecting survivors to healing possibilities.

Philadelphia Trans Wellness Conference
mazzonicenter.org/trans-wellness
Large annual healthcare conference.

Transgender Care Listings
transcaresite.org
Healthcare professional database.

Trans-Health
trans-health.com
Archive of health resources.

Healthline
healthline.com
Nice collection of Transgender Resources.

Trans Healthcare
transhealthcare.org
Surgeon database.

T-Vox

t-vox.org

Information and resources.

TransAdvice

transadvice.org

Peer-based live transgender support chat.

Law and Policy

National Center for Transgender Equality (NCTE)

nctequality.org

Social justice organization dedicated to advancing the equality of transgender people through advocacy, collaboration, and empowerment.

Sylvia Rivera Law Project

www.srlp.org

Collective organization founded on understanding that gender self-determination is inextricably intertwined with racial, social, and economic justice.

Transgender Legal Defense & Education Fund

transgenderlegal.org

Transgender legal resources.

Gay & Lesbian Advocates and Defenders (GLAD)

glad.org

Rights organization that has achieved scores of legal victories to end discrimination based on sexual orientation, HIV status, and gender identity and expression.

National Center for Lesbian Rights (NCLR)

nclrights.org

Non-profit, public interest law firm which litigates precedent-setting cases at the trial and appellate court levels; advocates for equitable public policies affecting the LGBT community.

Press for Change (PFC)

pfc.org.uk

Political lobbying and educational organization for all transgender people in the United Kingdom.

National LGBTQ Task Force

thetaskforce.org

Organization that builds the grassroots power of the LGBTQ community.

Transgender Law & Policy Institute (TLPI)

transgenderlaw.org

Organization dedicated to engaging in effective advocacy for transgender people.

Transgender Law Center (TLC)

transgenderlawcenter.org

Civil rights organization advocating for transgender communities.

TGI Justice Project

tgijp.org

Trans Justice Funding Project

transjusticefundingproject.org

Legal and financial resources.

Immigration Equality

immigrationequality.org

Advocacy for LGBTQ immigrants.

ACLU

aclu.org

LGBT Bar

lgbtbar.org

The Williams Institute

williamsinstitute.law.ucla.edu

Think tank on law and public policy for sex and gender minorities.

Lambda Legal

lambdalegal.org/know-your-rights#transgender

Human Rights Campaign

hrc.org

Race and Ethnicity

Black Trans Advocacy
btac.blacktrans.org

Trans Women of Color Collective
twocc.us

TransLatin@ Coalition
translatinacoalition.org

LULAC
lulac.org/programs/lgbt

Bienestar – Transgéneros Unidas
bienestar.org

Asia Pacific Transgender Network
weareaptn.org

National Black Justice Coalition
nbjc.org

El/La Para TransLatinas
ellaparatranslatinas.yolasite.com

Youth and Students

Gender Diversity
genderdiversity.org

Campus Pride
campuspride.org

TransYouth Family Allies
imatyfa.org

PFLAG
pflag.org

TransKinds Purple Rainbow
transkidspurplerainbow.org

Trans-Parenting
trans-parenting.com

Gender Spectrum
genderspectrum.org

Workplace Advocacy

TransTech Social Enterprises
transtechsocial.org

Transgender at Work
tgender.net

National Gay & Lesbian Chamber of Commerce
nglcc.org

Out & Equal
outandequal.org

Pride at Work
prideatwork.org

Transgender Community of Police and Sheriffs
tcops-international.org

Trans Educators Network
transeducators.com

General Resources

Transgender Life
tglife.com
Resources maintained by Brianna Austin.

Transgender Map
transgendermap.com
Resources maintained by Andrea James.

Susan's Place
susans.org
Resources, forum, and wiki focusing on trans women.

TransPulse
transgenderpulse.com
Resources and archive.

TG Forum
tgforum.com
Dedicated transgender forum.

FTM Magazine
ftmmagazine.com
Resources and news for transmasculine people.

Hudson's FTM Guide
ftmguide.org
One of the original comprehensive sites.

Julia Serano
juliaserano.com
Resources maintained by author and activist.

Marci Bowers, M.D.
marcibowers.com
Resources maintained by trans surgeon.

Glossary

A

acromegaly: Metabolic disorder caused by the presence of excessive growth hormone. It leads to enlarged body tissues, including bones of the skull.

Adam's apple: Prominent protrusion in the front of the neck formed by the angle of the thyroid cartilage containing the larynx. Adam's apples produce distinctive laryngeal lumps in adult men.

alar rims: Wing-like portions of the nostrils that normally flare slightly outward.

androgenetic alopecia: Common genetic form of hair loss in both men and women. This condition was formerly known as *male pattern baldness.*

anterior: Before or in front.

anterior neck approach: Reduction of the thyroid cartilage or Adam's apple through an incision in the front of the neck.

anterior open bite: Open space between the upper and lower anterior or front teeth. It is often caused by the thrust of the tongue, although thumb sucking in childhood can also be at fault. With this condition, the back upper and lower teeth meet, but the front teeth do not meet.

antihelical rim: Cartilage just inside the outside rim of the ear's pinna.

arch bars: Metal strips wired to the teeth to help stabilize the jaws during fracture repairs. They are also used to keep the upper and lower dental arches together after orthognathic surgery.

aspiration: Suction removal of fluid and cells from a cavity with needle and syringe.

asymmetry: Lack of proportion between two parts that would normally have a similar appearance and structure.

Avitene: Special collagen agent applied to control bleeding during surgery.

Avodart (dutasteride)**:** Oral hair restoration medication that works by preventing the conversion of testosterone to dihydrotestosterone (DHT), which causes male pattern baldness.

B

benign masseteric hypertrophy: Abnormal overgrowth of the masseter muscle, the thick rectangular muscle at the side of the face that helps close the jaw.

benign prostatic hyperplasia (BPH): Highly prevalent disease of older men whereby the prostate experiences unregulated nonmalignant growth.

bicuspids: Any of eight teeth located in pairs on each side of the upper and lower jaws directly in front of the molars, behind the cuspids. Also known as *premolars.*

blepharoplasty: Surgical reshaping of the upper or lower eyelids by removing and/or repositioning excess skin and fat.

blood coagulation study: A laboratory procedure to determine if a patient's bleeding time is normal or prolonged.

(bony) osteotomy: Surgical cutting of bone. A necessary procedure for shortening, lengthening, or otherwise reshaping a bone or its alignment.

brow bossing: Prominent bony ridge extending across the male forehead above the eyes. Brow bossing is a distinctive feature of a male skull that must be reduced to achieve a feminine look.

brow lift: Known also as a *forehead lift,* this procedure is used to elevate the brows to a normal height, especially in females. As such, it removes deep worry lines across the forehead. In facial feminization, it's usually completed after recontouring the frontal bone. During FFS, the procedure helps provide additional correction for sagging eyebrows.

buccal mucosa: Mucous membrane or lining of the inside of the cheek, continuous with the same membrane under the tongue's surface and the floor of the mouth. It is involved in mucous secretion.

C

cancellous bone: Spongy bone areas that make up the bulk of the bone's interior, surrounding the marrow. It lies adjacent to, and inside, the cortical bone, the extremely hard, dense outer skeletal shell.

cartilage: Tough, rubbery tissue found throughout the body. It helps form various facial features such as the ears and nasal tip. Cartilage acts as a shock absorber, reducing the friction between bones at the joints.

central incisors: Paired central teeth in the front upper jaw *(maxillary)* and lower jaw *(mandible)* for biting and chewing.

cephalogram (cephalometric radiographs): Precise radiograph of the skull that shows the relationships of the facial components. Doctors rely on the precise scientific measurements of cephalograms to plan surgical maneuvers during facial feminization and orthognathic procedures.

closed rhinoplasty: A rhinoplasty approach in which the surgeon enters the nose through the nostrils to reposition and remove cartilage and bone. Although this technique doesn't offer the doctor as much freedom to move as an open rhinoplasty, it provides many reshaping possibilities. The incisions (and scars) are also completely hidden afterward.

columella: Portion of the nose between the nostrils. When hanging downward in relationship to the alar rims, it is referred to as a *hanging columella.* Fixing this sagging condition involves reorienting the columella upward. The initial incision during an open rhinoplasty is made through the columella.

complete blood count (CBC): Yields information about a patient's underlying health by examining various blood components, including white cells, red cells, and platelets. Abnormally high or low counts may indicate a disease that might prohibit or need to be addressed before surgery.

comprehensive metabolic panel: Blood analysis of electrolytes, sugar (glucose), fluid levels, and kidney and liver function. Complete metabolic panels are often ordered prior to facial feminization surgery to rule out underlying medical conditions such as diabetes.

concave: Hollowed or rounded inward.

conchal cavity or bowl: Shallow conch shell-shaped formation inside the outer ear. Composed of skin–covered cartilage, it funnels sound toward the ear canal.

condyle: Rounded projection at the end of each bone that anchors the muscle ligaments and interacts with adjacent bones as a hinge.

convex: Curved or rounded outward.

coronal incision: Incision from ear to ear across the top of the head.

cricoid cartilage: Cartilage that rings the trachea below the thyroid cartilage, providing attachment for various other cartilages, membranes, and ligaments involved in opening and closing the airway. It also helps in producing speech.

cricoid–thyroid approximation: Surgery to alter the pitch of the voice involving the two main cartilages of the voice box: the thyroid and cricoid cartilages. In FFS, they are tightened through an incision on the front of the neck in an attempt to remove the lower pitches.

cuspids: Also known as *canines,* the cuspids have thin, bladelike crowns that are used for cutting food. They lie adjacent to the four front teeth in the dental arch on each side.

D

dental arch: Curving shape created by the normal arrangement of teeth in both the upper and lower jaw.

dermis: Thick layer of skin consisting of fibrous and elastic tissue. Directly under the epidermis or top layer of skin, the dermis contains nerve endings. The sweat glands, hair follicles, and blood vessels lie in the deeper subcutaneous tissue.

dihydrotestosterone (DHT): Chemical in the scalp that is believed to contribute to male pattern baldness in men. It shrinks hair follicles until they no longer produce visible hair. Some of today's hair medications work by inhibiting DHT.

donor area: In hair transplants, the area from which the hair follicles will be removed. Typically located at the back of the head where hair is genetically more permanent. Hair grafts taken from this area are moved to the area of hair loss, known as the *recipient area.*

Doppler: Ultrasound imaging technique to monitor the behavior of a moving structure, such as blood pulsating through the vessels or the heart beating.

dorsal: Reference to the back or posterior of a body part. May also refer to the upper surface.

dorsal hump: Bump on the ridge of the nose, which is characteristic of many men.

dorsum: Refers to back or posterior. It may also refer to upper surface, such as the vertical ridge along the top of the nose.

E

edema: Swelling of any organ or tissue due to an accumulation of excess lymph fluid. This retention can be caused by any number of health issues, including surgery.

electrocardiogram (EKG, ECG): Records the electrical activity of the heart. By producing various waves or patterns, it yields important information about the rate and regularity of your heart and the presence of abnormalities such as muscle damage.

electrolysis: Elimination of unwanted hair using electrical current aimed at the root. The number of sessions depends on many factors.

endoscope: Optic instrument illuminated to visualize the interior of a body cavity or organ. Available in many lengths, for various parts of the body, endoscopes can reach otherwise inaccessible areas because of their flexibility. Many surgeries today are performed endoscopically. The scope is placed through small keyhole incisions and creates less body trauma than open surgery.

epidermis: Outermost layer of the skin, which forms a waterproof, protective wrap over the entire body. Dead epithelial cells, which migrate from the deeper layers to the surface, make up the epidermis. They are eventually sloughed off in minute particles, such as dandruff and dust.

epiglottis: Elastic lid flap that guards the entrance to the glottis, the opening above the vocal apparatus of the larynx, so food doesn't go down the trachea during swallowing.

epistaxis: Nosebleed.

ethmoid air cells (ethmoid sinus): Numerous thin-walled cavities situated above the upper parts of the nasal cavities and between the orbits. They are part of the paranasal sinuses, or air-filled spaces within the bones of the face that lighten the skull.

F

facial feminization surgery (FFS): Collection of surgical procedures to increase the femininity of the human face. These surgeries alter various bony and soft tissue structures.

fiber optics: Process of visualizing internal organs or cavities using glass or plastic fibers to transmit light through a special tube that reflects a magnified image. Fiber optics give endoscopes the illumination power doctors need to explore the nooks and crannies of the body through a small incision.

fistula: Abnormal passage from an internal organ to the body surface or between two internal organs. Fistula can have many causes, including injury, infection, and congenital defects.

follicular unit (FU): A naturally occurring bundle of hairs. This bundle typically contains between one and three hairs.

follicular unit excision (FUE): A type of hair transplant that involves removing individual follicular units one at a time in their naturally occurring groupings

follicular unit transplant (FUT): The hair restoration technique whereby hair is transplanted in naturally occurring groups of one to four hairs.

forehead lift: Procedure to remove deep worry lines across the forehead and that can be useful to lift sagging eyebrows to a more feminine shape. It's usually completed after recontouring the frontal bone during facial feminization surgery.

Frankfort horizontal plane (line): Horizontal line passing from the highest point of the ear canal through the lowest point of the anterior orbital rim of the eye. Surgeons use it to establish a line of reference.

frontal sinus: Generally paired air-filled cavities within the frontal bones above the bony orbits that help lighten the skull. They're part of a honeycomb of mucous-secreting cavities in the skull.

G

galea: Tough, fibrous layer in the scalp between the occipital and frontal muscles of the scalp.

geniohyoid muscle: Narrow muscle in lower jaw involved in pulling the lower jaw down.

gingiva: Part of the soft tissue lining of the mouth that surrounds the teeth and seals them. When healthy, it is coral pink in color. When inflamed, it is red.

gingivitis: Inflammation of the outermost tissue, the gingiva, of the gums. If left unchecked, it may lead to periodontal disease.

glandular: Pertaining to a gland.

Golden Mean: Mathematical means of quantifying the proportional relationship between the whole and its parts. The most beautiful examples in nature, architecture, art, and anatomy always exhibit the Golden Mean ratio of 1.618 to 1.0.

H

hair follicle: Tiny tube within the skin made up of epidermal cells that produce and contain the root of a hair shaft.

hematoma: Swelling filled with clotted blood that develops within an organ or soft tissue such as subcutaneous tissue. Caused by a break in a vessel. Hematomas are rare, but still problematic complications of surgery.

high–density polyethylene: Thermoplastic material known for its durability and safety. It is used in many products, including medical prosthses such as MEDPOR.

horizontal ramus: Horseshoe-shaped portion of the mandible or lower jaw. It connects with the vertical ramus in the back of the jaw at the mandibular angle.

hyaluronic acid: Natural substance found throughout the body, particularly in skin and soft connective tissue. It transports essential nutrients, hydrates the skin, and acts as a cushion and lubricating agent. Synthetic forms of hyaluronic acid are being used to correct many facial disorders.

hydroxyapatite: Bone filler in its synthetic form, hydroxyapatite is a naturally occurring mineral in the body composed of calcium and phosphate. It gives bones, teeth, and similar structures their rigidity.

hyperpneumatization: Overdevelopment of air cavities such as the frontal sinuses.

I

iliac crest: Bony top ridge of the pelvis or hip.

induration: Hardening of tissue, particularly the skin, due to inflammation or swelling.

inferior alveolar nerve (or mandibular or lower jaw nerve): Receives sensation from the lower teeth, gums, lower lip, and chin.

infraorbital nerve: Branch of maxillary or upper jaw nerve that receives sensation from the lower eyelid, side of the nose, and upper lip and teeth.

intermaxillary fixation: Process by which upper and lower metal arch bars are secured to each other after the jawbones are repositioned.

K

keratin: Fibrous protein that is the main structural constituent of hair and nails.

keloid: Specific overgrowth of a scar resulting from an injury such as a cut. Varying in color, from pink to dark brown, keloids can appear either as a firm rubbery lesion or shiny fibrous nodule at the site of healing.

L

labial sulcus: Furrow between the lip and gum.

larynx: Organ in the neck above the trachea that produces sound. Also known as your *voice box*.

lateral: To the side.

lateral mound: The protrusion along the frontal hairline, on average 3.75 to 4.0 cm from the midline *widow's peak.*

lateral orbital rims: Bony or skeletal outside rims of the eye socket.

LeFort I osteotomy: Surgical approach to the upper jaw that relies on separating the dental arch of the upper jaw from its bony attachments and repositioning it.

lip reshaping: Procedure for changing the shape of the lip. It can be used to either reduce the vertical height of a male upper lip so that it looks more female, or to make the lips fuller by augmenting them.

long face syndrome: Facial appearance characterized by a long, narrow middle face and excessive upper tooth show.

M

malar: Pertaining to the cheek or cheekbone.

malar prominence: Cheek prominence.

malocclusion: Misalignment of the lower and upper teeth to each other.

malpositioned: Positioned incorrectly.

mandible: Lower jaw.

mandibular angle: Angle behind the lower teeth where the vertical and horizontal portions (rami) of the lower jaw meet.

mandibular nerve: *See* inferior alveolar nerve.

masseter muscle: A muscle at the back and side of the face. One of the strongest muscles in the face, the masseter assists with mastication or chewing.

maxilla: Upper jaw.

medial: Toward the midline of the body.

MEDPOR: High-density polyethylene implants for facial and/or skull surgeries.

mental nerve: Sensory nerve that receives sensation from the chin and lower lip.

mental protuberance: Bony triangular tip of the chin.

mentalis muscle: Muscle in the chin area that raises the lower lip to express doubt or displeasure. It also helps provide closure of the lips.

mesial–buccal cusps: Pointed ridges on the molar teeth that are toward the front and side.

mesial–buccal grooves: Corresponding depressions in the molar teeth.

methyl methacrylate (Lucite): Self-curing plastic injected under the temporalis muscle at the temporal fossa of the skull, or on the bone to augment the forehead and/or its depressions. It hardens into a permanent, non-carcinogenic material that weighs about the same as bone. It can be penetrated by normal X-rays.

molars: Largest and furthest back teeth used to grind food, especially meat.

N

nasal cavities: Paired large air-filled spaces behind the nose that condition the air as it enters the respiratory tract.

nasal notch: Depression at the top of the nose where it joins the forehead.

nasal septum: Partition dividing the left and right nasal cavities in the nose. It is composed of cartilage, bone, and mucous membrane.

nasal supra area: On the dorsum of the nose about 1.2 cm above the tip.

neck lift: Surgery to tighten the skin and generally the underlying platysma muscles, a neck lift is usually performed in conjunction with a facelift, but sometimes can be done alone. Usually accessed through incisions around the ears and under the chin, it's key to rejuvenating an aging neck.

nonunion: Permanent failure in healing of a fractured or cut bone. A serious complication, it can occur if the fracture moves too much during healing or if there is a poor blood supply.

nostrils: Paired external openings to the nose.

O

oblique line: Slant, or any variation from the perpendicular or horizontal.

occlusion: Normal contact between teeth. Good occlusion occurs when the peaks of the maxillary (upper) fit snugly into the grooves of the lower mandibular (lower) teeth and vice versa when the teeth meet.

open rhinoplasty: Approach to nose surgery involving a small incision across the columella, the pillar between the nostrils, to first expose the nose, followed by other incisions inside. An open rhinoplasty is preferred for more complicated cases because it allows greater visibility for the surgeon.

orbital socket: Conical cavity in the front of the skull, housing the eyes and their appendages.

orchiectomy: Surgical procedure to remove one or both testicles, the major source of male hormones. Removal decreases testosterone production.

orthognathic surgery: Surgery to correct conditions of the jaw related to structure, growth, and disorders that orthodontics can't treat.

ossification: Bone formation. Process by which connective tissue or cartilage morphs into bonelike tissue.

osteotomy: Surgery to realign bones by cutting and repositioning them.

otoplasty: Surgery to change the appearance or prominence of the outer ears. Otoplasty involves pinning back the *pinna* or external structure, reshaping the cartilage, and possibly reducing the earlobes.

outer cortical layer: Dense outer layer of bone, which provides a shell for a more porous cancellous inner bone.

P

panorex radiography: Full 180-degree anterior view X-ray of upper and lower jaws, teeth, temporomandibular joints, and maxillary sinuses. Used to locate abnormalities.

patient controlled analgesia (PCA): Method of timed, self-administered pain relief.

pattern baldness: Genetic type of hair loss that typically develops in early adulthood. Both "male" and "female" patterns exist, with the type of pattern being unrelated to that actual sex of the patient. (In other words, the pattern is referred to as "male" or "female," regardless of the genetic sex of the patient).

periodontal disease: Chronic inflammation of the tissue layers that support the teeth. If not treated, periodontal disease can lead to tooth loss.

periosteum: Fibrous membrane that covers the outer surface of bones.

philtrum: Vertical groove in the center of the upper lip.

pinna: Also known as the *auricle,* the pinna is the visible structure of the ears. Made up of skin and cartilage, it helps direct sound through the ear canal.

platelet-rich plasma (PRP) therapy: Therapy that uses concentrated injections of a patient's own platelets to accelerate the healing process and encourage growth of various tissues.

posterior open bite: Malocclusion of the mouth in which the upper and lower front teeth meet when the mouth is closed while the back teeth do not meet.

prehairline: Area directly in front of the hairline or scalp.

premolars (bicuspids): Two transitional teeth between the molars and canines on both sides of the upper and lower dental arches. They are used for grinding.

prognathism: Jutting or abnormally long lower jaw that causes an "underbite" with the lower jaw and teeth overlapping the upper jaw and teeth in the front.

Propecia: Also known as *finasteride,* Propecia is an oral medication used for hair restoration. It works by preventing the conversion of testosterone to dihydrotestosterone, a chemical in the body that causes male pattern baldness.

R

radiograph: X-ray-produced photograph, generally of bone.

radiolucent: Materials that allow X-rays to penetrate with minimum absorption. Because of its radiolucent properties, for instance, methyl methacrylate is a very useful bonding material used in reconfiguring facial areas and bone.

radix: Round top of the nose, just below the forehead between the skeletal sockets of the eyes.

ramus: Small branchlike structure extending from a larger one. The lower jaw comprises the vertical ramus, which intersects perpendicularly at the back of the jaw with the horizontal ramus.

retrognathism: Facial abnormality in which the lower jaw is abnormally short and recedes or is positioned behind the upper jaw. When the jaws meet, this situation causes an "overbite."

rhinoplasty (nose job): Normally used to improve the function and/or appearance of the nose, this procedure can be integral to facial feminization. In FFS, a rhinoplasty involves reducing the structure to give it feminine proportions to harmonize with the rest of the face.

rhytidectomy: Also known simply as a *facelift,* this cosmetic procedure produces a more refreshed appearance. Major surgery involves smoothing wrinkles, removing excess facial skin, and tightening underlying muscle.

rongeur: Heavy-duty forceps with a sharp-edged, scoop-shaped tip used to remove small pieces of bone or cartilage. In facial feminization surgery, a rongeur is employed to nibble off bits and pieces of thyroid cartilage in reducing an Adam's apple.

rotational or transpositional flap: Rotating flap of hair-bearing scalp from the temple area that is moved onto the forehead to reconstruct the anterior or front hairline.

S

sagittal split osteotomy: Surgical procedure to split the mandibular vertical ramus and move the lower jawbone either forward if it is too short or back if it is too long.

scalp advancement: Procedure to correct a receding masculine hairline by advancing the scalp forward.

scalp micropigmentation (SMP): Process where tiny points of pigment are applied to the scalp to replicate the natural appearance of real hair follicles.

scleral hemorrhage: Migration of blood into the sclera (white) of the eye.

sebaceous glands: Oil-secreting glands in the pores on the surface of the skin. They help remove old cells and keep the surface tissue lubricated.

secondary sexual characteristics: Traits that distinguish the two sexes, but are not related directly to their reproductive systems. In males, they include an Adam's apple, body and facial hair, a deepened voice, a larger skull with more prominent features, and broader shoulders. In females, these characteristics include smaller and shorter stature, a smaller skull with less prominent features, and a higher voice.

septal perforation: Hole in the nasal septum, caused by previous surgery, infection, disease, trauma, or drugs such as cocaine.

seroma: Localized accumulation of serum, or the clear watery plasma of the blood, that develops after surgery in tissues or organs.

seventh facial or cranial nerve: Seventh of twelve paired cranial nerves, the facial nerve controls the muscles of facial expressions, among other movements.

shock loss: Hair loss that occurs when the scalp undergoes a change or trauma that causes hair to shed in response. Most forms are temporary.

short face syndrome: Facial appearance characterized by a short middle third of the face, due in part to deficiency or undergrowth in the upper jaw's vertical length.

silicone rubber: Substance noted for its flexibility, resilience, and tensile strength over a wide range of temperatures. Used in many fields, such as medicine, for various purposes, including prostheses.

sliding genioplasty: Procedure whereby the chin is modified by cutting the lower jawbone *(osteotomy)* and moving the lower section.

sublabial sulcus: Shallow depression or groove between the lower lip and chin.

submental approach: Thyroid cartilage reduction approach that involves exposing the tissue through a cut of about 2.5 cm in the submental region. The submental region is the area under the lower jaw between the chin and the submental-cervical angle, the top of the neck.

submental-cervical angle: Angle at the top of the neck, going forward to the chin.

submental region: Area under the lower jaw between the chin and the submental-cervical angle, the top of the neck.

supraorbital: Upper rim of the eye socket.

sutures: Stitches that hold skin, muscle, and other tissue together after surgery or an injury. Sutures come in two types: *absorbable*, meaning they break down harmlessly over time, and *non-absorbable*, meaning they must be removed manually if on the skin surface.

symmetrical: Aesthetically pleasing balance between two like features. Opposite parts of the face have symmetry when they are balanced and equal to each other.

T

temporal fossa: Depression on the side of the skull just above the cheekbones behind the lateral orbital rims. Containing the temporalis muscle, one of the strong muscles used in chewing, the temporal fossa benefits from augmentation when it is depressed.

temporal points: Feature of a hairline that frames the face at the sides below the temples. In men it connects the hairline to the sideburns of the beard. In women it tapers away to create face-framing *tendrils*.

temporalis muscle: One of the major muscles responsible for raising and retracting the lower jaw as in chewing. Located on the lateral or side of the skull, the temporal muscle is engulfed by a strong fibrous covering, known as the *temporalis fascia. See* temporal fossa.

temporomandibular joint (TMJ): Joint of the jaw, formed by the upper temporal bone of the skull and the lower jaw or mandible.

testosterone: Hormone responsible for secondary male characteristics such as facial and body hair, enlarged bony features, the Adam's apple, and sexual potency.

thyroid cartilage reduction: Surgery to reduce the appearance of the Adam's apple. It involves reducing the cartilage either through an incision behind the chin and under the lower jaw or a cut directly above the prominence on the neck.

tracheal shave: Often used incorrectly to describe the reduction of the male Adam's apple. Because the thyroid cartilage, not the trachea, is reduced by cutting, rather than shaving, calling this procedure a "tracheal shave" is inaccurate but common.

turbinates: Long, narrow spongy shell-shaped bones that protrude into the breathing passage of the nose. They help moisten air inhaled into the respiratory tract.

U

unilateral: One side.

upper lip reduction: Maneuver that uses a shallow excision of tissue below the nose to reduce the distance between the nasal base and the vermillion of the upper lip. It has the effect of lifting the upper lip upward and outward to produce a more feminine, fuller, and even younger effect.

upper lip philtrum: Groove or vertical indentation in the mid-upper lip. It stretches between two other vertical ridges from the top of the lip to the base of the nose.

V

vasomotor rhinitis: Non-allergic condition that results in a constant runny nose. Although the cause is unknown, it is often a result of a marked improvement in the nasal airway following surgery.

vermillion: Fleshy red portion of the lips.

vermillion border: Thin line of demarcation between the ruby skin of the lips and the flesh-tone skin of the face.

vertical ramus: Upright portion of the lower jaw that rises perpendicular to the horizontal ramus and up to the mandibular joint at the back of the lower teeth. The vertical ramus is a broad bony quadrilateral portion of the lower jaw.

vertical ramus osteotomy: Surgical cut in the vertical ramus of the mandible that sets back the mandible or lower jaw in cases of prognathism.

vertex: Area of the head at the top of the head that is usually covered by a hat. Also known as the *crown,* it is a typical location for early hair loss.

Z

zygomatic arch: Bony arch of the cheekbone extending back toward the opening of the ear on the side of the skull. The temporal fascia and masseter muscle are attached to its upper and lower border.

Index

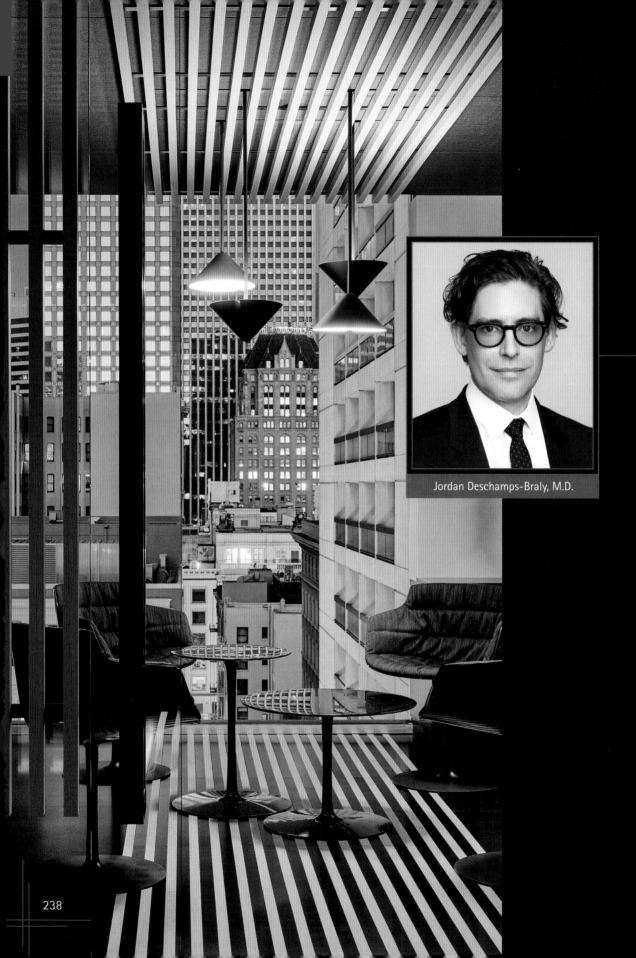

Jordan Deschamps-Braly, M.D.

About the Authors

JORDAN DESCHAMPS-BRALY, M.D., is a graduate of the University of Oklahoma, where he received his medical degree in 2005. As an undergraduate, he was a Phi Beta Kappa honors scholar. Dr. Deschamps-Braly completed his five-year surgery and plastic surgery residency in 2010. He held the position of chief resident from 2009 to 2010.

In 2010, Dr. Deschamps-Braly was accepted as a fellow in craniofacial surgery at Children's Hospital, Wisconsin, studying under Dr. Arlen Denny. Dr. Denny, like Dr. Ousterhout, was one of the very few Americans who traveled to Paris to study the techniques of craniofacial surgery under Dr. Paul Tessier.

Upon completing his craniofacial fellowship at Children's Hospital in Wisconsin, Dr. Deschamps-Braly, following the lead of Drs. Ousterhout and Denny, traveled to Paris where he pursued a fellowship in craniofacial and aesthetic facial plastic surgery under Dr. Daniel Marchac, a pioneer among surgeons in the International Society of Craniofacial Surgery.

In Paris, Dr. Deschamps-Braly performed pediatric craniofacial surgery at l'hopital Necker-Enfants Malades, the oldest children's hospital in the world. He also performed extensive aesthetic facial plastic surgery on women and men who traveled from all over the world seeking aesthetic facial surgery from Dr. Marchac's practice.

After completing his fellowship with Dr. Marchac, Dr. Deschamps-Braly traveled to Switzerland for a fellowship in orthognathic surgery at Dr. Obwegeser's clinic in Zurich. Dr. Obwegeser was the foremost pioneer in orthognathic (jawbone) surgery in the 1960s. He developed most of the surgical techniques now used for adjusting the upper and lower jaw structures. Those same techniques are now currently utilized in facial feminization surgery.

Dr. Deschamps-Braly is a member of the American Board of Plastic Surgery and a member of the International Society of Craniofacial Surgery. He holds full staff privileges at St. Francis Memorial Hospital in San Francisco. Dr. Deschamps-Braly has performed complex and demanding surgeries at locations in three different continents. He has coauthored and presented a number of major scientific papers, both nationally and internationally.

After several years searching for the right surgeon to be his successor, Dr. Ousterhout asked Dr. Deschamps-Braly to assume and continue his legendary practice in facial feminization surgery in June 2014. Dr. Deschamps-Braly is the only surgeon who has ever been trained in facial feminization surgery by Dr. Ousterhout.

Dr. Deschapmps-Braly may be reached at: **deschamps-braly.com**

⸻

DOUGLAS K. OUSTERHOUT, M.D., D.D.S., received his dental degree in 1961 and his medical degree in 1965 from the University of Michigan in Ann Arbor. Dr. Ousterhout continued at the University of Michigan as a resident in general surgery and completed his residency in plastic surgery at Stanford University Medical Center. From there he traveled to Paris to become the first American to assist Dr. Paul Tessier in the techniques of craniofacial surgery.

Upon his return to the United States, Dr. Ousterhout was certified by the American Board of Plastic Surgery in 1974, and then began his practice of plastic surgery in San Francisco. He is now retired from practice. He has fellowships with eighteen medical societies, including the American Society of Plastic and Reconstructive Surgeons, the American Association of Plastic Surgeons, the American Society of Aesthetic Plastic Surgery, and the International Society of Aesthetic Plastic Surgery, among others.

Dr. Ousterhout has served on the boards of several plastic surgical societies. He served as president of the American Society of Maxillofacial Surgeons from 1994 to 1995, and as president of the Pan Pacific Surgical Association from 1998 to 2000. Dr. Ousterhout has served on the editorial board of four different plastic surgery journals and is on the advisory committee for "Recommended Guidelines for Transgender Care," AEGIS.

Dr. Ousterhout is a clinical professor of plastic surgery at the University of California, San Francisco, and participates in a panel of experts at the Center for Craniofacial Anomalies. He has performed surgeries in many countries outside the United States.

Throughout his career, Dr. Ousterhout has presented dozens of major scientific papers, both nationally and internationally, and has published scores of scientific papers. His medical textbook, *Aesthetic Contouring of the Craniofacial Skeleton*, was published in 1991.

SARA WASSERBAUER, M.D., author of chapter 15, Hair Transplants, is a hair transplant surgeon with California Hair Surgeon. She has dedicated her professional career to the medical restoration of hair loss for both men and women. She believes that when performed properly, by a skilled and artistic surgeon, modern follicular unit hair transplants often have dramatic results for patients.

As one of the most experienced and accredited hair restoration surgeons in the United States, Dr. Wasserbauer has written several book chapters on hair loss, including most recently, "Eyebrows," "Scalp Micropigmentation," and "Women's Hair Loss." She has been featured on national television programs, including *The Doctors*, and speaks regularly at international medical conferences on hair loss and its surgical and medical treatment.

Dr. Wasserbauer was a Primary Investigator for the FDA's trial of the ARTAS Robotic Hair Transplant System; she also developed SYNSCALP, a new technology for scalp micropigmentation training, and was the first in the world outside of HairClone, to cryopreserve hair for future cloning treatments. She is past-president of the American Board of Hair Restoration Surgery and a Fellow of the International Society of Hair Restoration Surgery.

Dr. Wasserbauer completed her undergraduate studies at Dartmouth College in Hanover, New Hampshire, and earned her medical degree from the Medical College of Ohio in Toledo, Ohio. Her clinic is located in San Francisco, and in Walnut Creek, California, and she has several consult offices located around the Bay Area. Dr. Wasserbauer may be reached through her website: **www.californiahairsurgeon.com**